Claudia González, M.S., R.D., has served for six years as a spokesperson in charge of Latino affairs for the American Dietetic Association. She has more than ten years of experience working as a pediatric dietician in private practice as well as for government programs, and can be seen, heard, and read as a registered dietician through various media such as Univision, Telemundo, CNN, FOX, ABC, WFOR, *El Nuevo Herald, The Miami Herald,* and Hispanic Radio Network. Her nutrition columns can be found in *Shape en Español* magazine and on Univision.com and MiDieta.com. She lectures regularly on a variety of nutrition and health issues to national and international health organizations. Visit her Web site at www.latinosinshape.com.

Lourdes Alcañiz, M.A., is a journalist with over twenty-one years of experience writing, producing, and reporting on health-related subjects. She contributes regularly to magazines such as *Ser Padres, Avanzando, Su Bebé,* and *Su Familia.* She has reported on Latino health issues for Hispanic Radio Network, NBC-Canal de Noticias, CBS-UPI, Radio Voz, and Antena 3. A former Fulbright Fellow, she won an Emmy for news writing at Univision, and received the Radio and Television News Directors Foundation's Carole Simpson Fellowship. She is also the author of *Waiting for Bebé: A Pregnancy Guide for Latinas,* and won the 2002 Mariposa Award for Best First Novel (for her contribution to Kensington Publishers' bilingual collection, *Encanto*) at the Latino Literary Awards.

Gordito
Doesn't Mean Healthy

**What Every Latina Mother
Needs to Know to Raise
Fit, Happy, Healthy Kids**

Claudia González, M.S., R.D.,
and Lourdes Alcañiz, M.A.

Foreword by Univision anchor Giselle Blondet

BERKLEY BOOKS, NEW YORK

THE BERKLEY PUBLISHING GROUP
Published by the Penguin Group
Penguin Group (USA) Inc.
375 Hudson Street, New York, New York 10014, USA
Penguin Group (Canada), 90 Eglinton Avenue East, Suite 700, Toronto, Ontario M4P 2Y3, Canada
(a division of Pearson Penguin Canada Inc.)
Penguin Books Ltd., 80 Strand, London WC2R 0RL, England
Penguin Group Ireland, 25 St. Stephen's Green, Dublin 2, Ireland (a division of Penguin Books Ltd.)
Penguin Group (Australia), 250 Camberwell Road, Camberwell, Victoria 3124, Australia
(a division of Pearson Australia Group Pty. Ltd.)
Penguin Books India Pvt. Ltd., 11 Community Centre, Panchsheel Park, New Delhi—110 017, India
Penguin Group (NZ), Cnr. Airborne and Rosedale Roads, Albany, Auckland 1310, New Zealand
(a division of Pearson New Zealand Ltd.)
Penguin Books (South Africa) (Pty.) Ltd., 24 Sturdee Avenue, Rosebank, Johannesburg 2196,
South Africa

Penguin Books Ltd., Registered Offices: 80 Strand, London WC2R 0RL, England

This book is an original publication of The Berkley Publishing Group.

PRINTING HISTORY
Berkley trade paperback edition / April 2006

Library of Congress Cataloging-in-Publication Data

González, Claudia.
    Gordito doesn't mean healthy : what every Latina mother needs to know to raise fit, happy, healthy
kids / Claudia González and Lourdes Alcañiz ; foreword by Giselle Blondet.
        p.   cm.
    Includes bibliographical references.
    ISBN 0-425-20770-6
        1. Children—Nutrition—Popular works.   2. Hispanic American
children—Nutrition—Popular works.   3. Obesity in children—Prevention—Popular works.
I. Alcañiz, Lourdes.   II. Title.

RJ206.G56 2006
618.92'398008968—dc22   2005057112

PRINTED IN THE UNITED STATES OF AMERICA

10   9   8   7   6   5   4   3   2   1

PUBLISHER'S NOTE: Every effort has been made to ensure that the information contained in this
book is complete and accurate. However, neither the publisher nor the authors are engaged in rendering
professional advice or services to the individual reader. The ideas, procedures, and suggestions contained in this book are not intended as a substitute for consulting with your physician. All matters regarding your health require medical supervision. Neither the authors nor the publisher are responsible
for any loss or damage allegedly arising from the information or suggestions in this book.

While the authors have made every effort to provide accurate telephone numbers and Internet addresses
at the time of publication, neither the publisher nor the authors assume any responsibility for errors, or
for changes that occur after publication. Further, the publisher does not have any control over and does
not assume any responsibility for author or third-party Web sites or their content.

To all Latino families
working hard for a better future for their children

You will teach them to fly,
but they won't fly your flight.

You will teach them to dream,
but they won't dream your dream.

You will teach them to live,
but they won't live your life.

However . . .
in every flight,
in every life,
in every dream,
the road taught
will carry your footprints forever.

—Mother Teresa of Calcutta

Contents

Acknowledgments

First of all, we would like to thank our families, and especially our husbands and children, for their great patience and understanding during the creation of this book. There have been many hours spent in front of the computer and many more hours reading reports and scientific studies that we have needed to write *Gordito Doesn't Mean Healthy*. Our children, who range in age from two months to sixteen years, have understood us, respected us, and even brought us snacks or healthy dinners they have made themselves to "help Mami." Thank you, Carlos, Carolina, Cassandra, Adriana, Patricia, Alex, and Gabriela.

We want to thank too Rosa Alonso Leon, a nutritionist in Miami, for the hours spent reviewing the Latino pyramid for this book and for contributing her pertinent observations. Patricia Inda Icaza, a dietitian in Mexico City, who graciously reviewed the accuracy of the Mexican foods for the Latino pyramid. María Reyes, a nutrition and dietetics student at Florida International University, who helped with the preparation and tasting of the sample menus. Milagros Buero, a wonderful child behavior specialist, for all her guidance and advice; and María Jesús Cano and Luis Miguel Rufino for all their help with the book illustrations and Javier Pino for the design of the Latin food pyramid.

We also want to thank our editor, Christine Zika, and our literary agent, Judith Riven, for their great professionalism and help.

And a special thanks, above all, to all Latino children in the United States and worldwide, because you are the inspiration for this book.

Our greatest wish is for *Gordito Doesn't Mean Healthy* to contribute to making your child's future a healthier one.

Foreword

by Giselle Blondet

It's a privilege and honor to write the Foreword for a book I consider essential reading for Latino families.

Every day we see stories in the media about poor nutrition and childhood obesity in the United States. Latino children usually play a starring role in these sad stories because they're the most obese group in the country due to certain physical, cultural, and social characteristics they share. So many people have written books addressing proper nutrition and how to prevent childhood obesity, but until now not one of them has dealt with the specific problems Latino parents face.

Nutritionist Claudia González, an expert dietician I have collaborated with on many occasions, and Latino health journalist Lourdes Alcañiz have teamed up to write this book that's been missing from the shelves of so many Latino homes. Claudia and Lourdes are not only Latino health professionals, they're also mothers—three children for Claudia and four for Lourdes—who experience firsthand the daily challenge of providing their families with nutritious meals while at the same time working full-time. The experiences, advice, and practical menu suggestions they include in this book finally answer questions so many other Latino health books didn't. *Gordito Doesn't Mean Healthy* offers Latina mothers the knowledge they need to better understand what's really going on with their children's nutrition and the tools they need to live healthier lives, without forgetting what it means to be Latina. This book is a real gift for all of us because "we are too blessed to be stressed," and these two angels are taking out the stress related to our children's nutrition so we can relax and keep enjoying the adventure of motherhood.

Introduction

"Oh, *que lindo gordito,* what a cute, chubby baby, so strong and healthy!"

In Latino culture, this is one of the highest forms of praise for a mother. For many Latina mothers, a *gordito*—a chubby baby—and a healthy baby are synonymous. Same goes for most *abuelitas, tías, primas,* grandmothers, aunts, cousins—everyone in the entire extended Latino family. For a long time this way of thinking had some merit: Chubby babies indeed developed stronger immune systems and were better able to fight off infections. So, before the days of antibiotics and vaccines, a *gordito* baby had a better chance of survival. That's why generations of grandmothers and mothers were obsessed with making sure their children cleaned their plates at every meal. Eating a lot was nearly a guarantee for a child's survival.

But things have changed in recent decades in industrialized countries, including the United States. Nearly all children are vaccinated against known diseases. Antibiotics fight infections. Other medicines and medical equipment treat all kinds of illnesses. And there's no shortage of affordable food, available day and night, every day of the week.

The United States is home to the fattest children in the world, and a majority of them are Latino. *Gordito* doesn't mean healthy anymore; in fact being overweight is just the opposite. Overweight children are more likely to suffer diseases that will affect them for the rest of their lives. We're talking about diseases such as type 2 diabetes, high blood pressure, and high cholesterol. These problems will weigh heavily on a child's physical and psychological development and health well into the future.

As nutrition and journalism professionals, we've seen firsthand how obesity is affecting Latino children in the United States. And *como madres latinas*, as Latina mothers, we understand how confusing it can be for Latinas to decide what's best for their children. On the one hand, our culture tells us a chubby child is a healthy child; but on the other hand, the media continually bombards us with the dangers of obesity. In addition, most Latina mothers also work full-time, and when we arrive home completely *exhaustas*, worn out from a hard day's work, we have to clean, cook, and take care of the children. Even though the advice most media experts offer—eat better, exercise more—is correct, it's not that simple for Latino families who, at most, have three or four hours after work before it's time to go to bed. Cooking takes time; exercising takes time.

Also, Latino children have certain genetic, cultural, and social characteristics other children don't. Dozens of studies, investigations, surveys, and publications deal with the subject of childhood obesity, but few focus on Latino children and hardly any offer advice specifically for Latino parents. Consider this book a guide for Latino parents on how to create a nutritious diet and a healthy lifestyle for our children, without abandoning our *herencia latina,* Latino heritage.

The first part of the book explains what's really going on with nutrition and our Latino children and the risks our children face when they don't eat properly. You'll also read about the traditional Latino diet and how you can incorporate Latino flavors and ingredients into a healthy menu. The second part of the book provides practical solutions to common nutrition problems, as well as examples of foods, portions, and menus appropriate for children of all ages, from birth to nineteen years. The last chapters deal with the problems caused by eating disorders and obesity. And at the end, you'll find a resource guide with telephone numbers and addresses of organizations that can help you set your family on the road to a healthy life.

As Latina mothers, we know how difficult it can be to provide the best nutrition possible for our children. So we encourage you to put our recommendations into practice as a way to begin leading a healthier lifestyle. We assure you this is one of the best things you can do, not only for your children, but for *toda la familia*, the entire family.

—Florida, spring 2005

1

What's Happening to Our Children?

For generations, Latina mothers didn't worry if their children were overweight. Quite the contrary: Chubby babies were seen as healthy babies, whose mothers took good care of them and kept them *bien alimentados*, properly nourished. After all, parents figured as the boy or girl reached the teenage years, he or she would grow several inches, and the baby fat would melt away. Who hasn't heard stories about siblings, aunts, uncles, or cousins who were chubby as children, hit puberty, grew like weeds, and poof . . . no more extra pounds!

The fact of the matter is, generations of Latino parents have been less worried about whether their children were overweight than whether they were *comiendo bien*, getting enough to eat. This belief that obesity is actually something healthy and desirable continues among many Latinos today.

The problem is that things have changed from the good old days. Before, overweight children were still likely to grow up into healthy adults because the foods they ate and their daily activities helped to burn off the fat. In past generations, fast food wasn't such a big part of the diet, portions were smaller, and children walked to school and then played outside around the neighborhood with the family. Nowadays it's much more likely an overweight or *gordito* child will turn into an overweight adult. Government statistics over the past thirty years show how much society's waistline is growing. Specifically, the data show people who are classified as being of normal weight have gained just a few pounds over the years. However, people who are classified as overweight have gotten much, much heavier over the same time period. In other words, *gorditos* are now more *gordito* than ever. In fact, an obese child today has a 70 percent chance of being an obese adult; that likelihood goes up to 80 percent if one or both of the child's parents are obese. This is particularly important for the Latino community, because our children are more overweight than any other group in the United States.

As you probably know, being overweight is not good for your health. Overweight people have higher cholesterol levels, are more likely to suffer a heart attack, and, among Hispanics, are more likely to develop type 2 diabetes (which can result in blindness, kidney problems, and even limb amputations).

As the title of the book says: An overweight or *gordito* child is *not* a healthy child. Just the opposite. An obese Latino child is almost guaranteed to be an overweight adult. Moreover:

- The younger a child becomes obese, the more obese he'll become as an adult, that is, the more amount of weight he will have as an adult. The amount of extra weight in adulthood seems to be linked to when childhood obesity started.

- The sooner a child becomes obese, the sooner he'll become obese as an adult, that is, he will be obese earlier in his adulthood.

- Weight gain during and after puberty increases the likelihood children will become obese adults.

Obese children suffer even before they become obese adults. Being an overweight child carries with it a whole series of physical and psychological problems that only get worse as the years go on. For example, six out of every ten obese Latino children have type 2 diabetes; a high percentage of them suffer orthopedic problems, and a good number of them have psychological difficulties because they're often ridiculed by their friends. *Gordito* no longer means healthy.

The obesity epidemic among our children has really taken off in the past few years. There have always been overweight children; I've treated many of them as a pediatric dietician. But only a few years ago, I began to notice a radical change in my practice. Three out of every five patients were obese children, and most of them were Latinos. Of course, because I speak English and Spanish, I was more likely to see Hispanic patients. Still, the number of overweight Latino children I was treating alarmed me. So I did a little research, and the statistics confirmed that what I was seeing in my office was happening across the country.

According to a health and nutrition study carried out between 1999 and 2002, the number of obese children in the United States has tripled since 1980. There are now 9 million children whose weight is above normal. And the numbers are even more alarming for us Latino parents, because our children are the most obese of all, from preschool right through to adolescence.

Race	Children 2–5 years		Children 6–11 years		Teens 12–19 years	
	Overweight	*Obese*	*Overweight*	*Obese*	*Overweight*	*Obese*
Latinos	26.3%	13.1%	38.9%	21.8%	40.7%	22.5%
African-Americans	23.2%	8.8%	33.7%	19.8%	36.8%	21.1%
Whites	20.8%	8.6%	28.6%	13.5%	27.9%	13.7%

A study comparing obesity rates among teenagers in fifteen industrialized countries showed children who live in the United States are the most overweight, far heavier than the others. So if Latino kids are the most overweight in this country, that makes them the most overweight in the world.

Imagine how we'd feel if there were an infectious disease that afflicted one out of four of our children. We'd do something right away to eliminate this disease and protect our children. The consequences of being overweight can be just as severe, and in some cases even more damaging than a typical infectious disease. What I am trying to point out with these figures is that this is a grave problem. Being an overweight child does not show health anymore but a strong possibility of being sick or getting sick in the future.

But why do Latino children seem to be more susceptible to obesity? The problem is so severe that several studies have explored the issue. Early results of these studies show a mix of cultural, genetic, and social factors contribute to a high rate of obesity among Latinos.

Cultural Factors

We Latinos take great pride in our culture. For generations, we've followed our own traditions and trusted our own way of looking at the world. If truth be told, many of us would rather trust *que nos mamás, abuelitas, y suegras dicen*, what our mothers, grandmothers, and mothers-in-law say than what our pediatricians or dieticians tell us. Why? Well, who wouldn't take the word of a female relative who has successfully raised four, five, six, even seven healthy children!

WHY IS THE BELIEF THAT *"BEBÉ GORDO, BEBÉ SANO,* A FAT BABY IS A HEALTHY BABY," SO ROOTED AMONG LATINOS?

The idea that carrying a few extra pounds meant being healthy made a lot of sense for many centuries. In the past food wasn't as plentiful as it is today, so a child with a good weight, or who was even heavy, had a good chance of surviving if food suddenly became scarce. Scientists have proven children with a normal weight develop stronger immune systems compared to skinny children (although recent studies have shown that obesity can also damage a child's immune system).

Historically obesity has been viewed as a sign of wealth and power. If you go to a museum with classic paintings you'll see that the noble and wealthy beauties the painters of the past chose as subjects almost always had some extra pounds. Even in religious paintings, the little angels and Baby Jesus are, for the most part, *gorditos*. In general, the healthy infant was represented by painters as an overweight child.

This relationship between excessive weight and health is still alive in the minds of many *mamás latinas*, Latina mothers. You may have heard someone in your family talk about the difficult times when food was scarce and people went hungry before migrating to the United States. These were times when losing a baby during the first months was common. The idea that babies need to *comer*, "eat up," to be healthy has been passed down for generations of Latina women, from grandmothers to mothers to daughters. We Latina mothers have a great deal of respect for what our mothers think. Grandmothers always have something to say about how we should feed and raise our babies. And if a grandmother says, "*El bebé tiene que comer más*, Feed the baby, he is not eating enough," sometimes that could be more influential than the recommendations of our baby's pediatrician.

In addition, there is the high value Latino culture places on motherhood, on *ser una buena madre,* being a good mother, and on caring for our children properly. What better way to show how much we love our children than having a well-fed child, a child who can prove it by being a little *gordito*? The charts the pediatricians show us that rank our children in the 85th to 95th "percentile" (see charts in the Appendix) give us a lot of pride rather than worry. It's as if they represent grades of our job as mothers: "Look, our baby is among the best! We must be good mothers!"

Also it must be said that until recently, many pediatricians didn't consider obesity among infants a problem serious enough to try to prevent. Generally, pediatricians only began to fight obesity in alarmingly overweight children. The American Pediatric Association has just recently recommended its members check for obesity among infants during routine visits.

OBESITY PERCEPTION AMONG LATINO PARENTS

In short, a great majority of Latina mothers don't think there's any reason to worry about an infant, especially one younger than two, who begins to show signs of obesity. It's not thought of as an illness that needs to be treated as soon as possible because of the dangerous consequences it can bring.

The idea that Latino parents believe *gordito es saludable*, obesity is healthy, has been proven by various studies. In one of the more recent surveys, nearly half of Latino mothers and fathers said their children weigh just about the right amount, when in fact those children were either obese or clearly overweight. The problem is that parents who don't consider their children's weight a concern don't do anything about it, nor do they have their children participate in programs to prevent or control obesity at this age.

NO COME NADA, HE WON'T EAT A THING

I can't tell you the number of times I've heard Latino parents complain: "*No come nada*, my child won't eat a thing." The pediatricians I've worked with confirm that's one of the greatest worries Latino parents have.

But I've learned when Latino parents say, "My child won't eat," they are not really saying that. What they really mean is "My child isn't eating as much as I think he should be eating" or "He doesn't seem to be eating as much as he used to." Of course, the child may indeed be eating less than he did during a growth spurt. "My child won't eat" hasn't anything to do either with the child's weight. Often Latina mothers will worry about how much a child is eating, when the baby's weight is normal, or maybe even a little high. This attitude is tied directly to the belief in our culture that a *gordito* baby is a healthy baby. But insisting that a child eat when he doesn't want to can create many more problems than solutions in the future.

Several studies over the past few years have shown a relationship between how a mother feeds her baby and how much the baby weighs and what food he likes. These studies have also made a connection between how a mother feeds her baby and the baby's ability to regulate how much food he eats, according to his inner hunger clues. In other words, when we force our babies to eat when they're not hungry, or when we use food as a reward or *para calmar al bebé*, to calm our babies, the child doesn't learn to distinguish between hunger and fullness. Food is no longer seen as a source of nutrition; it becomes a source of emotions. A baby who sees food as a reward or as a means to calm down will not be able to differentiate between when he's bored or fidgety and when he's really hungry. Babies are born with the ability to regulate their appetites. So by teaching our babies that food has other purposes, we're spoiling our babies' own ability to know when they're full and even when they're not hungry in the first place.

THE MORE TIME SPENT IN THE UNITED STATES, THE MORE LIKELY TO BE OVERWEIGHT

Another factor that makes Latino children more likely to be obese has to do with where they live. Recent immigrants to this country are less likely to be overweight. One study on this topic showed that immigrants begin to gain weight ten years after living in the United States because after a while Latinos abandon their traditional native diet, which is considered healthier than what's eaten in the United States. For example, people who were born and raised in Mexico and later move to the United States often continue to follow a diet that contains less fat and more fiber, vitamins, calcium, potassium, and magnesium, while people of Mexican descent who were born in the United States eat foods that aren't as healthy. On the other hand there are also some Latinos who abandon their healthy diets soon after they arrive because they feel "eating American" is a way to absorb their new culture faster.

Soft drinks and sugared drinks exemplify a product Latino children drink too much of while in the United States. The explosion of childhood obesity in the past years coincides with the increase in the consumption of soft drinks and sugared drinks by children. Children are drinking them three times more. One reason is that schools have signed contracts with soft drink makers to allow vending machines on campus in exchange for part of the profit (to be spent on supplies, computers, repairing the school, etc.). Some states prohibit these vending machines from being set up on the school campus and other states are considering similar restrictions. Just to give you an idea: One twelve-ounce can of soda contains ten teaspoons of sugar and a two-liter bottle of soda contains forty teaspoons of sugar and loads of calories without any nutritional benefit (these calories are known as empty calories).

Children can't help but be confused if during health class they hear how bad soft drinks and junk food can be for them, then when they walk out into the hallway, they see vending machines selling these same drinks and food.

Despite all the cultural factors that contribute to childhood obesity among Latinos in the United States, they're not entirely responsible for the problem. Scientists have discovered other causes that play an equally important role in the obesity epidemic among Latino children.

Genetic Factors That Contribute to Obesity in Latino Children

In the past fifteen years we have seen a huge increase in obesity in the United States among children and adults of all races. For a while, the consensus was that this increase in weight was attributable to an increase in food consumption, especially foods high in fat and sugar and calories, as well as a lack of exercise. While this is undoubtedly part of the problem, it's not the entire problem. Scientists are now beginning to consider genetics as a factor.

Genes are made up of chromosomes, which we inherit from our parents—half from Mother and half from Father. Chromosomes, and the genes they make up, are found in every cell in the human body (except red blood cells) and they determine our physical traits. Investigators have discovered that one of the physical characteristics we can inherit is obesity, especially Latinos.

The first study to take a look at the genetic component of obesity took place more than a decade ago in the United States scientists compared the levels of obesity between twins (who have the same genetic makeup) raised in the same family and between twins raised in different families. They discovered the differences in weight were minimal. Today there are many more studies that clearly show the relationship between genes and obesity.

Experts now believe genes play a major role in two out of every five cases of obesity. This connection between genes and obesity is even more pronounced in Latinos, which is to say that many Latino children are born predisposed to become overweight. And it's not just obesity that has a genetic basis. Type 2 diabetes is a disease related to obesity that disproportionately afflicts Latino children, and it too has been found to have a genetic cause that's passed on more frequently between Latino generations than other races.

When you combine the predisposition to be overweight with a diet high in calories, fats, and sugars, and then you mix in a lack of exercise, what you get is precisely the obesity epidemic we're seeing today in our children.

GORDITO PARENTS, *GORDITO* CHILDREN

Obesity is passed on from one generation to the next in many Latino families. The experts have proven it: Children who have one overweight parent are likely to be overweight themselves; children who have two overweight parents are twice as likely to suffer from the same problem as they grow older.

It's common for Latino children to have obese parents; after all, Latinos are the most overweight group of people in the United States. It's a fact that the mother's weight during pregnancy plays a role in determining whether the baby will have a tendency toward obesity during childhood.

According to a recent study done among obese pregnant mothers, children whose mothers were obese during the first three months of pregnancy had twice the chance of being overweight between two and four years of age. Also, children at that age who are overweight are much more likely to become overweight adults.

GESTATIONAL DIABETES AND INFANT OBESITY

Gestational diabetes (diabetes that occurs during pregnancy) is much more common among Latinas than the rest of the women in the United States. This type of diabetes happens when the hormones secreted by the placenta make it more difficult for insulin to work properly. As your body digests food, insulin carries the glucose from the food to individual cells throughout your body. That's how the cells get the fuel they need to work. If the insulin doesn't carry the fuel to the cells, the fuel (glucose) sits in the bloodstream and instead is passed on to the baby. This is similar to feeding your baby candy all day long. The result is that the baby gets very big. Besides the problems you'd expect trying to give birth to a large baby (C-sections, birth complications, etc.), the baby will probably be obese during childhood.

It seems pretty clear that we Latinos have a genetic tendency toward obesity. But why? There are several theories that seem to explain why our ability to gain weight was at one time an evolutionary advantage for our ancestors. The food storage theory goes like this: During times of plenty, when there was a good harvest or a good hunting season, our

Latino ancestors stored up much of the food they ate in fat, so in times of want, when the harvest or the hunt wasn't so good, they had their own "fuel" in reserve, right on their bodies. This genetic mechanism that helped our ancestors survive has now turned against us Latinos who live in times of perpetual plenty. We can eat pretty much what we want, where we want, when we want. Add to that a sedentary lifestyle and a lack of exercise and there's no way we can burn off all those calories our bodies are inclined to store in the first place.

Investigators have had some success recently studying how genetics affects animals. For example, scientists have discovered that certain rats that lack a particular gene don't get fat no matter how much they eat! It'll be a while before there's a genetic way to battle obesity in humans, but it's important to understand that obesity among Latinos isn't only caused by eating too much and not exercising (although that's obviously part of it). There are other factors that may be out of our control that make it more difficult for Latino children to maintain a healthy weight.

This is not to say Latinos should take on a fatalistic attitude, the *fatalismo* so common in our culture: "This is how we were born and there's nothing we can do about it" or "*Dios nos lo envió,* God sent it to us." On the contrary, it's precisely because we are predisposed to be overweight that we must take control and take the proper steps to make sure our genetic heritage doesn't manifest itself. And believe me, there are plenty of things you can do to keep your own and your child's obesity genes in check. This book will provide you with the tools you'll need to prevent and control obesity in your children.

Social Factors

Beyond the cultural and genetic factors that make Latino children more likely to be obese, there are several other social circumstances that affect the Latino population and that don't make things easier.

LACK OF HEALTH INSURANCE

We Latinos have less health insurance coverage than any other ethnic group in the United States. One-third of the Latino population doesn't have any health insurance at all. In part, this is because many Latinos don't make enough money to pay for private insurance but at the same time earn too much to qualify for Medicaid. Also, many Latinos work for companies that have few employees. Those companies aren't legally required to offer health coverage to their workers. The result is that many Latino children don't go to the pediatrician on a regular basis. According to official statistics, one of every four Latino children between the ages of six and eleven hasn't been to the doctor in the last year. Without medical supervision, there's no way to catch obesity in its early stages or to prevent its consequences, such as type 2 diabetes, a disease that affects a disproportionately high number of Latino children.

WORKING MOTHERS

Two of every three mothers who have young children work. Out of those, three-quarters work more than thirty hours a week. And Latina mothers are no exception. A household where both parents work is the norm these days, not the exception as it was a few years ago. Working full-time takes time away from other activities, such as going to the supermarket, cooking, exercising, or even being at home when the kids return from school. Many Latino families can't afford to have one of the parents give up work to stay home to care for the children.

This family circumstance is so common today, the effects can be seen in what our children eat, how they eat, and how much they eat. Fast food or frozen dinners are *rápido y barato*, quick and cheap, so many families depend on them when there's no time to cook. However, these types of meals tend to have more fat, salt, and sugar than meals that are considered healthy. For example, a hamburger, french fries, and a soft drink have between 700 and 1,000 calories, which is more than half the calories a five-year-old child needs in an entire day. Think about it: one meal, half a day's worth of calories.

So what's the alternative if the majority of Latino parents need both mother and father to work? There are ways to ensure your children live a healthier lifestyle, whether you leave every morning for work or not.

TELEVISION AND OBESITY

Television is considered one of the main culprits of childhood obesity, according to several studies. Unfortunately, Latino children watch television as much as or more than any other group in the United States: at least four hours a day or more.

Television promotes obesity for several reasons:

- The time children spend seated in front of the television is time not spent exercising.

- It's common to eat snacks or sweets while watching television. Therefore, the more television children watch, the more snacks and sweets they eat.

- Children's television programs include plenty of advertising about food products. Children who see more food commercials eat more of the food they see in the commercials, certainly more than the children who haven't seen the ads.

Something as simple as removing the television from your children's room can help them to lose weight. Children who have televisions in their rooms are some of the most overweight, according to another study.

LACK OF EXERCISE

A sure formula to gain weight is to consume more calories and exercise less. More than 60 percent of all children in the United States don't play any sports or get any outdoor exercise during the week. Our children are among the ones who get the least amount of weekly exercise in the United States.

Hispanic parents often complain that it's difficult for them to transport their children to recreation centers, they don't have time to take them, or the activities cost too much. Also, nearly half of the Latino parents interviewed for one study said they felt more comfortable having their children play at home instead of out in the yard or at the park down the street.

How Doctors Treat the Problem: Cultural Barriers

There's another factor Latino parents should keep in mind: the interaction you have when you take your obese child to a pediatrician who isn't familiar with the Latino culture.

Latino doctors, or doctors who are familiar with the Latino culture, may treat patients differently from other doctors. It's common among Latino patients and doctors to start the visit off with a handshake and small talk before getting to the heart of the matter. We Latinos also have the custom of *sonreir más,* smiling more, looking each other in the eyes, and leaving less space between us when we talk. The absence of these signals when we're talking to a doctor who doesn't know our culture could be interpreted as a lack of interest in our children. Nevertheless, it's important for us Latinos to understand there are different ways of treating patients, and none of these factors necessarily means the pediatrician won't give us the proper care we deserve. In the American culture, efficiency and punctuality are valued. If a doctor only has ten or fifteen minutes with each patient, he's going to want to make the most of that time and that may be why he gets straight to the point at the beginning of the visit.

Don't forget, as we explained at the beginning of this chapter, the perception of what obesity means may be different for Latino parents and others. It's common for a Latina mother to take her well-fed, perhaps chubby child to the pediatrician because "*No come nada,* he just won't eat a thing." The doctor may ignore this complaint and tell the mother her child is overweight and the child's diet must change or health problems will crop up in the future. What the doctor may not understand is that to the Latina mother, a chubby baby is a healthy baby and that the best thing she can do for her child is to get him to *comer más,* to eat more. This scenario would play out much better if the doctor would explain that chubby doesn't mean healthy and that the child has a much greater chance of being obese into adulthood and of getting sick. A simple recommendation to see a dietician or to read this book would bridge much of the cultural gap. In fifteen minutes, a doctor just can't provide the tools and knowledge necessary to treat a case of childhood obesity.

What's required is a change of attitude and perspective on the part of both the parents and the doctor. In the following chapters, you'll find the reasons why it's important to keep your children from becoming overweight and what you can do to help them follow a healthy diet.

2

Is My Child Obese?
Health Risks of
Childhood Obesity

Many of the children I treat at my practice are sent to me by pediatricians who have found they are not only obese but also have diabetes. The first step is to explain to the parents exactly what changes will have to be made in their child's life: a better diet, more exercise. Many of those parents say, "Great. When will my child recover from diabetes and return to a normal lifestyle?" They're shocked when I tell them, "Never, diabetes is a disease that never goes away, it's for life." These parents think diabetes is a disease that's treated and then disappears, like an earache or a sore throat. But diabetes and many other illnesses related to obesity don't ever go away. Sure, you can control it with a proper diet and exercise, but in most cases, patients can't go back to their old way of living because some organs have been damaged for good and can't be repaired.

I wish we had known before that we needed to watch Matilda's weight. You see, her father is diabetic, so is my mother and her aunt. But we didn't know that she could be diabetic so young. She is only ten!
                                                                    —Marta, thirty years old

Other parents who come to my practice know their children are obese, but they don't think the dangers from obesity will affect their children now. They believe health problems related to being overweight only appear in adulthood, and if their child loses some extra pounds before then, everything will be okay. Unfortunately, this is not so. Overweight children not only have a higher risk of becoming sick adults but also of being sick children as well. As we'll see in this chapter, recent studies have shown obese children, especially obese Latino children, are already suffering a whole series of illnesses that previously were only thought to affect adults. And many of these diseases, such as diabetes, damage the body in irreversible ways.

The information you read in this chapter may make you uncomfortable. The fact of the matter is that these statistics must be taken seriously because the obesity epidemic among Latino children today is real. But information is one of the most potent weapons you have to fight this problem and keep your children from becoming obese in the first place. In the following pages, you'll learn how childhood obesity works, how Latino children are affected, and ways to better understand what your pediatrician is telling you about your child's weight.

Is My Child Obese?

You might think the easiest way to tell if children are obese is to look at them. The answer is yes and no. It is true that certain stages of obesity are obvious to the eye. But we Latinos have a different understanding of what it means to be overweight than pediatricians do. In general, Latino parents think a chubby child, especially a young one, is a healthy, well-fed child.

> Mi mamá, *my mother, always gives me a hard time with my son's weight: "¡Este niño está muy flacucho! This boy is too thin!" But according to my pediatrician his weight is perfectly fine. Sure, he's not one of these chubby babies, nor was his father when he was his age, but he is healthy and happy, and to me that's what counts.*
>
> Hortensia, twenty-five years old

There are various ways to measure obesity, but the most common you'll hear from your doctor are "percentiles" and body mass index (BMI).

During a visit to the pediatrician, your doctor will weigh and measure your child and then tell you he is in a certain "percentile" (25, 50, 80, etc.). Right after that, you and just about every other mother will ask: "What does that mean?"

Using the BMI table (see page 20), the pediatrician will determine where your child's height and weight fall in comparison with other children of the same age and characteristics. Here's an exaggerated example to help you understand. Imagine two groups of children side by side. In one group you've got the Batusi, one of the tallest ethnic groups on the planet. In the other group, you've got Pygmies, one of the shortest ethnic groups in the world. The average height of a Batusi is seven feet (more than two meters). The average height of a Pygmy is four feet three-fourths of an inch (1.38 meters). So what would happen if a Batusi family adopted a Pygmy? How would the tall parents know their short child was healthy and growing properly? Comparing the rest of the tall Batusi children with the shorter adopted Pygmy wouldn't make much sense because they're so different. But a Batusi pediatrician with a chart that showed the average growth rate of Pygmy children would have an accurate reference point. That's what growth tables are.

However not all children of the same race, age, and sex are the same height, even if all of them are perfectly healthy. Most will be about the same height, but some will be taller and others shorter. Growth tables reflect these differences among children of the same demographic group, age, and sex. Scientists have spent years collecting data on children's heights and weights and have created a scale that goes from 1 to 100. The results are read as a percentage.

So when your pediatrician measures your child at a certain age and then refers to the growth chart, the result is a comparison of the height of your child to other children of the same group, age, and sex. For example, if the pediatrician says your child is in the 50th percentile, that means 50 percent of the children of the same group, age, and sex are shorter than your child, and the other half of the children in the same group are taller. Your child is right in the middle. If, say, your child is in the 70th percentile, that means 70 percent of the children in that group are shorter and 30 percent are taller. The lines on the table separate the different percentiles. And the same thing goes for the weight comparison table. If your child is in the 50th percentile, half of the children in the same group, age, and sex weigh more, half weigh less. Each time you take your child to the doctor, the pediatrician will mark the spot on the growth and weight charts showing where your child is at that visit. As your child gets older, you can see the changes in development over the years. You will find the growth charts in the Appendix.

Other growth charts measure BMI. The BMI correlates height and weight to determine whether a person is overweight; knowing the person's weight alone isn't enough. Tall children generally weigh more than shorter children, even though they may all have the same amount of body fat. The BMI is calculated using a pretty simple formula. (If you're good at math you may even be able to do it without a calculator), or the *Gordito Doesn't Mean Healthy* Web site will calculate it for you. Check the Resource Guide. The BMI Resource can be calculated using kilograms and meters or pounds and inches, whichever is easier for you. Use the BMI to situate your child in a growth table and see where your child is compared to other children. If your child is above the 85th percentile on the weight chart, that's obese. The BMI number will also help you compare your child to these established markers:

BMI RANGE

BMI	Level of obesity
Up to 27	Normal
27–30	Slightly obese
30–40	Moderately obese
More than 40	Severely obese

To calculate the BMI using kilograms and meters you need to know your child's weight in kilograms and height in meters. For example, let's suppose your child weighs 40 kilograms and is 1.22 meters tall (one meter, 22 centimeters). Multiply the height by itself ($1.22 \times 1.22 = 1.48$). Then divide your child's weight by this number (1.48), that is: $40/1.48 = \mathbf{27.02}$. This is the body mass index for your child. The formula is BMI = weight in kilograms / (height in meters)^2.

If you're more comfortable using pounds and inches, you need to know your child's weight in pounds and height in inches. If your child weighs 88 pounds and is 48 inches tall, you begin the same way: Multiply the height by itself: $48 \times 48 = 2304$. Now, divide the weight by that number (88/2304) and multiply the result by 704.5. Again: $88/2304 = 0.038 \times 704.5 = \mathbf{26.9}$. That's the BMI of your child. The formula is BMI = weight in pounds / (height in inches)$^2 \times 704.5$.

This might all seem a little complicated and confusing, but it's important for your child's health. First of all, if you don't understand BMI and percentiles when talking to your pediatrician, the information won't do you any good. Second, it's a good tool for you to use in your own home to help determine whether your child is overweight.

In the example we gave, the child had a BMI of 27, meaning normal body weight, but nearly entering the slightly obese category.

How We Get Fat

Accumulating fat on our bodies makes us fat. Many organs and body systems are involved in this process. In the case of Latinos, several studies have shown that some systems work differently in our bodies than they do in other ethnic groups. Unfortunately, that difference makes us more likely to gain weight. To get a better understanding of which foods and behaviors your child should avoid, let's take a general look at what our bodies do with the foods we eat.

For your car to run, you've got to fill it with gasoline. The same goes for your body's cells. They need fuel to carry out their jobs: to pump blood, pull air into the lungs, etc. But cells can't use the food we eat as fuel until it's first converted into smaller units. The process by which food is converted into fuel our cells can use is called digestion. Digestion transforms the foods we eat and the drinks we consume into smaller nutrients the body can use as fuel to power our cells and create new ones.

Everything we eat can be classified into three general categories, according to what they're made of: carbohydrates, proteins, and fats. The body uses each one of these groups of foods in a different way. In Chapter Three you'll find various lists of foods and the categories they belong to and you'll learn just how important it is to eat the right portions to maintain a healthy diet. Now let's take a look at just what the body does with each of these groups of foods and what the difference is between eating a peach (carbohydrate) and eating a steak (protein).

CARBOHYDRATES

Carbohydrates are found in foods such as tortillas, pasta, cereal, sweets, fruits, and vegetables. Some foods that have carbohydrates also contain fiber, which is the part that isn't digested. Fiber helps keep the intestines functioning properly. Without fiber, you end up constipated.

After carbohydrates have been chewed and they enter the stomach, the decomposition process continues, and they're reduced to even smaller pieces as they mix with the gastric juices. Eventually, they're broken down into basic particles called glucose. The intestines absorb the glucose and it passes into the bloodstream.

Glucose is a type of sugar; it's the type of fuel our cells depend upon most. Blood distributes glucose to cells throughout the body. Glucose is important because it's the only element (except in cases of sustained hunger) that provides nourishment to our nervous system (the brain, spinal column, and nerves). If the nervous system doesn't have enough glucose, other parts of the body—such as the heart and lungs—stop working. For the nervous system to work at an optimal level, its cells need to have a steady glucose supply. In order for cells to be able to use glucose, they need something else provided by the pancreas: *insulin*. Insulin is like a key that opens the door to the cells, allowing glucose to enter and be used as a fuel. The pancreas secretes different amounts of insulin depending on how much glucose is in the bloodstream.

The amount of insulin in the bloodstream and its effectiveness play an important role in childhood obesity among Latinos. Several studies have shown that many Latino children are genetically predisposed to having difficulties secreting the proper amount of insulin in the bloodstream and often their cells can't use the insulin to unlock the doorways to allow glucose in.

PROTEINS

Proteins are found in foods such as red meat, fish, cheese, eggs and vegetable proteins such as nuts, soy, and quinoa. When proteins are digested, they're broken down into amino acids. Just like with glucose, the blood distributes amino acids throughout the body. Cells use amino acids to construct new proteins that keep bones, skin, and muscles working properly.

FATS

Fats are found in foods such as butter and oil. Most fats we eat are made of *triglycerides*. Triglycerides are one of the body's storage forms for fat. When the body digests triglycerides, they're broken down into two elements: glycerol and fatty acids. Glycerol and fatty acids can be used as fuel by all the cells in the body. However, the brain mostly relies on glucose.

WHAT HAPPENS WHEN WE EAT TOO MUCH AND OUR CELLS DON'T NEED ANY MORE FUEL?

The answer to this question is critical to understanding why we get fat. What our body doesn't use right away isn't tossed out, it's stored. Storing extra food as fat for later use helped our ancestors survive for thousands of years. During prehistoric times, and for a long time after that, food wasn't as readily available as it is now. Sometimes our ancestors would go days without eating before they found more food. But the cells in their bodies needed fuel every day, they couldn't just shut down and wait until the next successful hunt. So to make sure cells had enough fuel in reserve during these times of want, our bodies converted stored fat into fuel.

The three groups of nutrients (carbohydrates, proteins, and fats) are each stored in different ways. Imagine your child eating a hamburger and french fries. Whatever the body doesn't use right away as fuel is stored in the following ways:

- Carbohydrates (the bread, lettuce, tomato, and the potatoes): The glucose that the cells haven't used right away is stored in the liver and in the muscles as *glycogen*. Glycogen is a compound formed by a chain of glucose (think of many, many glucose molecules linked together like the beads of a necklace). This compound is the first "extra fuel tank" the body uses when it needs more energy. The rest of the glucose that's not stored as glycogen is transferred to specialized fat-storing cells called *adipocytes* (which also play an important role in childhood obesity among Latinos).

▪ Proteins (the meat): Cells use the amino acids in protein to make new protein. If cells already have all the proteins they need, what's left over is used as energy if needed. But after that, any extra protein is stored as fat in the adipocytes.

▪ Fats (the oil used to fry the french fries and fat from the meat): Fat is broken down into glycerol and fatty acids. If they're not used as energy right away, they are immediately stored as triglycerides in the adipocytes.

As you can see, everything we don't use as energy is stored as fat. That means it's not only the fats we eat that turn into fats but also carbohydrates and proteins that aren't used for energy in the hours after we've finished eating. If your child doesn't eat much fat but does eat big portions of carbohydrates (bread, pasta, sweets) or proteins (red meat or chicken), his body will store all the extra food as fat.

Losing weight is the same process in reverse. If we reduce the amount of food we eat and increase the amount of energy we burn through exercise, our body will first use up all the food we've eaten for energy, and then turn to the "extra fuel tanks" for more. Remember that the glucose level in the bloodstream has to remain constant for the brain and the rest of our body's organs to work properly. The body first uses glucose stored in the liver and muscles as glycogen and then starts to break down the triglycerides stored in the adipocytes to make more glucose and more energy.

ADIPOCYTES

Adipocytes are cells whose specialty is storing fat. Under a microscope, an adipocyte looks like a cell with the nucleus pushed to one side because the rest of the space is used to store fat (see Figure 2,

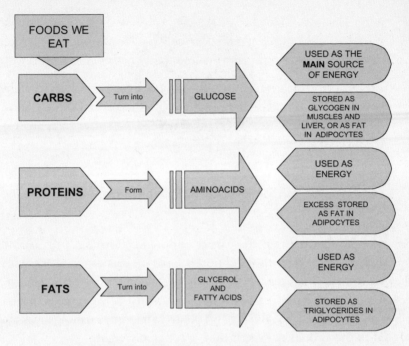

Figure 1: **Food Transformed into Energy and Fat.**

page 26). Compared to other cells, they have a pretty long life span. Adipocytes don't divide in two as other cells do, and when a person begins to gain weight adipocytes accumulate fat until they seem ready to explode. If we continue to eat too much, and there is not enough space inside the adipocytes to store the extra fat, our body will send out a signal to the reserve adipocytes, which are not completely formed yet, that they need to spring into action and begin to store all this extra fat. That's how we form new adipocytes to store more and more fat.

We're born with a limited number of adipocytes. When a child gains a lot of weight and gets fatter during the first few years of life, the child will have larger adipocytes, but not more of them. Between four and seven years of age, there's a period called *adiposity rebound*. During this normal process, the number of adypocites does increase.

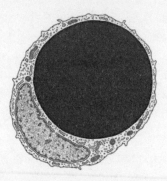

Figure 2: **Adipocyte (The Black Area Is Stored Fat)**

Research has shown that the earlier children go through this period, the greater the chance those children have of becoming obese when they're adults. During adolescence, body fat increases again, and it's distributed in different parts of the body. Girls have a greater probability of gaining weight during this stage, while boys usually accumulate fat in the abdomen, even if they don't gain weight.

These different stages are really important for us Latinos to keep in mind. What determines the number of adipocytes a baby has when it's born is how much weight it gains in the womb during the last three months before birth. Latina women are more susceptible to diabetes, and to diabetes during pregnancy (gestational diabetes), than any other ethnic group. One of the side effects of diabetes during pregnancy is that the baby gains a lot of weight, and heavier babies are born with more adipocytes. Even without the problems of gestational diabetes, statistics show Latino children are born heavier that most other children.

Scientists are looking into what factors cause the adiposity rebound period between four and seven years old, and why this period starts earlier in some children than others. Diabetes during pregnancy seems to be one of the factors in having an earlier onset of the adiposity rebound.

Also recent studies have shown that *where* a child accumulates fat can affect that child's health in different ways. Fat around the stomach area is not the same as fat that accumulates on the hips or thighs. Latino males between the ages of twelve and nineteen are more obese than any group in the United States, and most of them have an excessive accumulation of fat in the stomach area.

BODY SHAPE: APPLE OR PEAR

Fat that surrounds many of the organs in the abdomen and protects them is called *visceral fat*. Fat that accumulates below the skin is called *subcutaneal fat*. Subcutaneal fat has several functions, including keeping us warm. In the lower part of the body, all fat deposits are subcutaneal (buttocks, thighs, lower legs).

In men fat is found mostly in the abdomen, while in women fat deposits are usually found from the waist down. People who have a lot of belly fat are said to have an "apple" body type. People whose fat is found in the buttocks, hips, and thighs have "pear" body types. According to research our body types are inherited: Pears tend to have pear offspring, apples produce apples.

Having an apple or pear body type is more than just a matter of looks. It can also have health implications. During the past few years, studies have shown that visceral body fat, that found within the abdomen, is much more than an extra source of energy; it plays a key role in how our bodies function. Visceral fat, or the adipocytes that make it up, secretes various chemical compounds, some of which can harm the body. Adipocytes found beneath the skin (subcutaneal fat) apparently do not have this capability.

Visceral fat has been related to various health risks, such as high cholesterol, glucose intolerance by the cells, and the pancreas secreting too much insulin.

These factors are important to Latino children for two reasons: Latino children have more fat in the abdominal area than other children. Second, too much visceral fat is related to two illnesses that affect obese Latino children: insulin resistance and metabolic syndrome.

Fortunately, there is good news too. These studies have also shown visceral fat is also the easiest to lose through exercise.

Consequences of Obesity for the Physical Health of Children

You probably already know what happens to adults who are obese: They're at risk for high cholesterol, diabetes, heart attacks, arteriosclerosis (hardening of the arteries), and joint pain. All these risks have been well documented for years. But investigators have been shocked to learn recently that these same physical problems are already present in many obese Latino children. That means being obese not only makes children more likely to be obese as adults; they're also likely to suffer the same physical problems obese adults do, regardless of their youth. The consequences of obesity for children go beyond the physical; they also affect them emotionally and socially.

> I know that my life will change completely if I can lose some weight. I will feel much more confident in my appearance. I feel bad now. I don't like the way I look and I'd rather stay home than go out.
>
> —Laura, fourteen years old

What you're about to read isn't supposed to alarm you. It is, however, supposed to focus your attention on a problem that, perhaps for cultural reasons ("a gordito baby is a healthy baby"), we Latinos don't necessarily take too seriously.

INSULIN RESISTANCE

The health problems obese Latino children develop usually start with something called insulin resistance. Insulin is a hormone or chemical compound secreted by the pancreas. More specifically, special cells in the pancreas called beta cells produce insulin.

You'll recall that the job of insulin is to unlock a "door" in the cells so glucose (fuel) can enter. Insulin resistance happens when cells don't "hear" the insulin as it knocks on the door asking the cell to let in the glucose. When the cells don't respond, the glucose sits in the bloodstream and blood sugar levels skyrocket. When the pancreas detects high levels of sugar in the blood, it naturally produces even more insulin, hoping eventually the cells will hear the knocking and let in the glucose.

This process will work for a while. But over time, the beta cells in the pancreas get worn out from producing so much extra insulin. Eventually they begin to fail. This is the beginning of type 2 diabetes, or diabetes caused by obesity. Beta cells can't regenerate or reproduce, which means when they die, it's for good.

Insulin resistance is hereditary, and not long ago, scientists identified the gene that causes insulin resistance in people of Mexican origin. The problem with insulin resistance in children is that their beta cells, which are supposed to make insulin for their entire lives, can't keep up with all the extra work and fail quickly.

More Latino children have type 2 diabetes than any other group of children in the United States. Researchers are trying to figure out why. Latino children have higher levels of insulin than non-Hispanic white children to begin with (an indication that their pancreas has to work harder to deal with blood sugar); add to it overeating and lack of exercise and it's more likely that this genetic trait will appear. One study reports that one of every three obese Latino children who has at least one diabetic parent, grandparent, or sibling is insulin resistant, and in many of those, their beta cells are already failing. Insulin resistance is also more likely in these cases:

- when the child's mother had diabetes during pregnancy (common among Latina mothers);

- when fat accumulates in the abdomen (obese Latino children have much more visceral fat);

- during adolescence because the body is going through a natural stage of development where there's more insulin resistance than normal.

Insulin resistance can be measured through a blood test after drinking a glucose mixture. Insulin resistance is one of the components of a condition known as metabolic syndrome, which affects many obese Latino children.

METABOLIC SYNDROME

Metabolic syndrome is a series of abnormal health conditions that indicate a high risk for developing heart problems and type 2 diabetes. Children are considered to have metabolic syndrome when they have three or more of the following abnormalities:

- *Abdominal obesity.* Fat that accumulates in the abdomen creates more health risks than fat that accumulates in other parts of the body.

- *Low HDL cholesterol.* You may have heard that people with "high cholesterol" need to take special care of themselves. Cholesterol is a type of fat that flows through the bloodstream and participates in many of our body's functions. HDL cholesterol is known as the "good cholesterol" because it helps remove the "bad cholesterol," or LDL, from the walls of the blood vessels.

- *Elevated triglycerides.* Triglycerides are a type of fat that circulates through the bloodstream too. They come from the fat in the

foods we eat and the fat we have stored in our bodies. When people are overweight or they eat more than they need to, triglyc-
eride levels go up. Triglycerides also travel through the body
attached to a lipoprotein. That's why they're also known as
VLDL (very low density lipoprotein).

- *High blood pressure, or hypertension.* This is the pressure the
  blood exerts on the walls of the vessels as it's pumped along by
  the heart. Arterial pressure depends on the amount of blood the
  heart pumps and the elasticity of the arteries and veins to accommodate more or less blood. The harder the heart has to work to
  move blood throughout the body, the higher the pressure. Fatty
  tissue requires a lot of blood to be maintained. So the fatter a person is, the more blood there is, and the harder the heart has to
  work to pump it through the body.

- *Glucose intolerance.* Glucose intolerance means blood sugar levels go up after eating, although not as high as in cases of diabetes.
  Glucose intolerance is related to insulin resistance (remember,
  that's when the cells don't "hear" the insulin knocking on their
  doors to let glucose in and the pancreas has to produce more insulin so it can knock louder). The next step is failure—partial or
  total—of the beta cells in the pancreas. Eventually glucose intolerance turns into diabetes.

Nine of every ten obese Latino children who have parents, grandparents, or siblings with diabetes suffer at least one of the characteristics of metabolic syndrome. Three of every ten actually develop
metabolic syndrome. The abnormalities most common among obese
Latino children are, in order: abdominal fat, low levels of "good cholesterol," and high blood pressure.

What this means is that obese Latino children *are already* suffering
health problems as a result of their being overweight; they've already
got an excessive amount of fat circulating in their blood, they've already got high blood pressure, and the beta cells in their pancreases are

already failing. In other words, obesity is making your child sick right now, you don't have to wait until adulthood for the effects to begin. In addition, when your children do grow up, they will also have a higher probability of suffering from high blood pressure, high cholesterol, diabetes, and all the health problems that these illnesses may bring (heart attacks, strokes, kidney and eye problems, etc.).

Type 2 Diabetes

Type 2 diabetes follows glucose intolerance. In cases of glucose intolerance, the cells in charge of making insulin may have begun to fail because they've been worked so hard trying to make more and more insulin.

As we've seen, without insulin, glucose can't get into cells and fuel them. So instead, it stays in the bloodstream. Some common symptoms of diabetes are:

- Frequent urination and persistent thirst

- Extreme hunger

- Weight loss

- Fatigue and irritability

Latino children are more likely than any other children to get type 2 diabetes. Many Latino adults have this disease, and children who are overweight and have diabetic relatives are more likely to get it. If the mother had diabetes during pregnancy, the probability is even greater.

Fatty Liver

This condition is an accumulation of triglycerides or fats in the liver. The liver performs an important function in the body: It filters the blood and regulates the levels of the majority of chemicals in it. It is also responsible for more than five hundred other essential body functions. A fatty liver generally doesn't have any symptoms, but can eventually degenerate into cirrhosis. Cirrhosis means the liver cells die and are so scarred they don't let blood through. There is no cure for cirrhosis of the liver.

GALLSTONES

The gallbladder is a small muscular sac that stores the bile produced by the liver. Bile is a greenish-yellowish substance that helps to break down the fats we eat. "Stones" form in the gallbladder when the bile is too concentrated. They can obstruct the passageway out of the gallbladder. When this happens, the gallbladder gets inflamed and can be very painful. Gallstones are common among people of Mexican origin.

APNEA

Apnea is a condition that impedes proper breathing during sleep. Apnea is often accompanied by snoring. When someone who has a lot of fat behind the soft palate falls asleep, the muscles relax and that fat can obstruct the airway. People with apnea can actually stop breathing when they fall asleep. As you can imagine, continually having your sleep interrupted by periods of apnea makes it difficult to get a good night's rest, and can interfere with school performance. Apnea also can result in high blood pressure and heart problems. This lack of rest can create all kinds of problems at school, from difficulty in concentrating to hyperactivity.

MENSTRUAL ABNORMALITIES

Obesity interferes with the way female hormones regulate the menstrual period. Girls who are overweight often enter puberty early: They get their periods earlier than normal and their breasts and pubic hair grow sooner. Menstrual cycles may be irregular or painful. Obesity also can cause infertility when it causes a condition called polycystic ovarian syndrome. Obese women have higher incidences of uterine, ovarian, breast, and gallbladder cancer.

ORTHOPEDIC PROBLEMS

Excess weight can cause the interior part of the tibia (one of the bones that run between the knee and the ankle) to develop abnormally. The legs become curved and there is a chance the child will have orthopedic problems or arthritis early in adulthood.

DARKENING OF SKIN IN BODY FOLDS AND CREASES (ACANTHOSIS NIGRICANS)

These are dark velvety patches that appear on the neck, the armpits, or in other places where the skin folds. These are common among children with insulin resistance. They aren't damaging to the skin itself, but when they appear they can be a sign that something else is wrong: insulin resistance.

Mental Health Consequences

If you've got a school-age child, you already know *gorditos* can be rejected by their classmates simply because of their physical appearance. Overweight children are often the subject of jokes, teasing, and isolation. When we parents say, "Don't pay them any mind" or "They'll get over it" or "*Mejor encuentra otros amigos,* Try to make some nicer friends," we're really not helping the problem. The majority of children and teenagers I see in my practice live with obesity as if it were a stigma, like some type of ranking that always places them beneath their peers. Obese children can be rejected at school, and that can in turn damage their self-esteem and in some cases even cause depression.

LOW SELF-ESTEEM

Self-esteem is how people view themselves. People with low self-esteem usually describe themselves in negative terms and don't think they're as good as everyone else. In the years leading up to adolescence, the love and approval children get from their families is vital to a healthy self-esteem. But the first years of adolescence are another stage. This is when the opinions of friends begin to matter as much as or more than what family members think. Teenagers gauge their self-esteem during this period by focusing outside their families. A teenager rejected because of obesity may have a low self-esteem that can continue into adulthood.

Teenagers who don't think much of themselves are sadder, spend more time alone, and are more nervous than their companions. Moreover, they're more likely to smoke cigarettes and drink alcohol. According to research, Latina girls in general have lower self-esteem.

NEGATIVE BODY IMAGE

Today's society places a very high value on a slim body. We're constantly inundated with images of fabulous models and movie stars, all with spectacular bodies that remind us how less-than-perfect the rest of us are. When obese children compare their bodies with these images or with the figures of more fit friends, they begin to form a negative body image. They may feel ashamed of their bodies and want to try to get thinner. Nine out of every ten children who are overweight are embarrassed about how they look and believe if they lost weight people would stop teasing them. Besides influencing self-esteem, a negative body image is the root of many other illnesses such as binge eating, anorexia (not eating), or bulimia (binge eating followed by vomiting to prevent weight gain).

DEPRESSION

In some obese children, the sadness and isolation that comes with be-ing rejected by friends can lead to depression. In the case of Latino children, they're already at a higher risk for depression. The most ex-treme cases of depression may end up in suicide.

Depression is a serious illness that involves chemical imbalances in the brain, and it must be treated. Nevertheless, we Latinos don't have much sympathy for mental illnesses. Instead we think it's about feeling tired or *tener nervios*, being nervous or sad. The truth is depression isn't something children can solve for themselves just by "trying to be happier." It would be similar to asking somebody with diabetes to "try to produce more insulin." Some of the symptoms of depression in-clude sadness, inability to concentrate, and changes in appetite and sleep patterns.

Social Health Consequences

Society places so much importance on physical appearance, many peo-ple are first judged based on how they look, even in academic environ-ments. The National Education Association conducted a study on rejection of obese children that showed "students who are overweight suffer constant prejudice, discrimination and harassment by their classmates."

NEGATIVE STEREOTYPES

The social rejection that overweight people suffer isn't only because they don't conform to what's considered a pleasing or beautiful body shape. There are certain ideas consistently associated with obese peo-ple. The assumption is that they don't possess self-control, they suc-cumb to temptation easily, and they're lazy. In other words, there's an entire stereotype applied to overweight people that makes life difficult for them very early on. One of my young overweight patients didn't ever want to go to the movies or watch television because overweight people are always presented as losers. One study showed overweight students were accepted to college less often than normal-weight students were, even though they had the same grades as their classmates.

DISCRIMINATION

Discrimination against overweight people begins at a young age and continues as the obese child grows older. And for overweight Latino children who are also trying to learn a new language and adapt to a new culture, this discrimination makes integration that much more difficult.

This phenomenon was proven in an interesting scientific investigation. Children of different social classes were shown photographs of obese children and photographs of children who had some type of visible physical impediment, such as a lost arm or facial disfigurations. The question was: Who would you like to be your friend? In every case, the overweight children were the last chosen as friends, even after the handicapped children.

SOCIAL EXCLUSION

Social development for children and teenagers depends on being accepted by peers and participating in activities with the rest of the group. Among Latino children, participating in school sports is a great way to build self-esteem and health, according to various studies (in addition to the benefits of weight control). Nevertheless, because of the extra weight they carry, many obese children don't have the agility needed to participate in games or other athletic activities that require physical exertion. So even though they want to join in, these children are left out. Besides the sadness, shame, and loneliness these experiences cause obese children, the fact of the matter is, when it happens over and over again, it can affect the child all the way through to adulthood.

Another thing to keep in mind is that obese children tend to be taller than their friends who aren't overweight. Because of their appearance, they're often considered more mature than they really are, and a level of behavior is expected of them that doesn't correspond to their age. This can also cause relationship problems.

Long-Term Consequences of Childhood Obesity

Plenty has been written about the health risks obese adults suffer, especially during the past few years as the obesity rate has skyrocketed in the United States. Many of those risks have their roots in childhood obesity. Below are a few examples, but there are many more:

- People who develop type 2 diabetes during infancy have much higher rates of heart and circulatory problems.

- Teenagers who have a body mass index higher than 30–40 have a much bigger risk of dying from heart and circulatory problems, even if they lose weight as adults.

- People who have elevated levels of cholesterol as children continue to have that same problem as adults.

Have no doubt, obesity in children, even when they're very young, is not a sign of good health. To the contrary, it's an indication that during infancy and in the following years they'll be at risk for various health problems as well as psychological and social problems that children who aren't obese don't necessarily have to deal with. In the case of Latino children, our genetic and cultural heritage makes the possibility of becoming obese in infancy even greater.

But don't give up hope. As bleak as this scenario looks, stopping and preventing obesity in your children isn't all that difficult. The first step: Learn about how obesity affects children and what its consequences are. You're already doing that by reading this book. And second, change your children's diet and lifestyle if you have to. The following chapters will help you achieve these changes.

3

Why a Healthy Diet Is Important for Children: Foods and What They Do

Sailors of centuries past feared not only storms at sea but also a mysterious illness called scurvy. This illness killed more sailors than all naval battles combined during the great sailing ship era. Scurvy caused bloody gums, bruised fingernails, breathing difficulties, and finally death. Many hundreds of years went by before an English doctor figured out that if sailors ate lemons during these long sailing ventures, they wouldn't get scurvy. Today we know that this disease and others were caused by the unbalanced diet sailors ate on long trips. The main problem was that they didn't eat fruits or vegetables. Scurvy is caused by a lack of vitamin C.

This is an extreme example of what can happen when a person

doesn't eat a balanced diet. But not eating the right foods can cause many problems; a child's development can really be harmed if certain nutrients are lacking during important growth stages.

A balanced diet gives us energy and the nutrients we need to carry out our daily activities. Essentially a balanced diet allows the body to work as it should and to regenerate itself. In addition children need a balanced diet so their bodies can create more new cells and muscles and bones. In other words, a balanced diet allows children to grow and develop properly.

In the following pages, you'll find out why you should give children certain foods to eat and what the differences are between foods. You'll also discover which foods contain the vitamins and minerals your child needs to grow and develop into a healthy adult.

Food Groups

Our body uses different foods in different ways, depending on the food's characteristics. Some foods are used as energy almost right away, such as carbohydrates. Other foods are used to regenerate tissues, such as proteins. Fats, on the other hand, are an important source of reserve energy. A balanced diet has specific proportions of each of these groups of foods, depending on the age and needs of your child. In the following chapters you'll learn what the appropriate proportions of these foods are for children ages zero to nineteen. Plus, you'll see a whole list of interesting and tasty menus. But before we start talking about foods, we should first focus our attention on an essential component of any balanced diet: water.

WATER

Water is necessary for life. If you've followed news of the recent exploration of other planets, you'll recall one of the great hopes for scientists is finding a planet that has or had water. That's because life prospers in environments that include water. Water facilitates the chemical reactions of life. In our bodies, cells take in energy and get rid of waste through water in order for our organs to work. Cells have water inside them and our tissues are bathed in water. In fact, about 60 percent of our body weight is water. Water allows us to get rid of waste through urine (that's the waste filtered by the kidneys) and through sweat (that's how the body regulates its temperature). To stay in top condition, our bodies need a certain amount of water every day. We may survive several weeks without eating, but barely three days without drinking; however, children—especially infants—can get dehydrated very easily.

Some of our required water comes from foods that contain it, such as fruits and vegetables. The rest comes from the liquids we drink, such as milk, soups, and sodas as well as from foods that turn to liquid inside the body, such as jelly, frozen yogurt, and ice cream. The amount of water children should drink varies according to age (see Appendix).

Water works best in the body when it's drunk unadulterated, just plain and simple water. Short of that, try to choose liquids made of 90 percent water, such as milk, soup, or the natural juices of some fruits. Some sodas contain caffeine, which increases urine production. That means that in the end, instead of taking in extra liquids, we actually lose more through urination after drinking caffeinated sodas. Sodas and other sugared drinks also contain a lot of sugar and other additives (one can of soda contains ten to twelve teaspoons of sugar). One of the best things you can do for your children's diet is teach them to drink a proper amount of water at an early age.

Something important to remember is that by the time we feel thirsty, we're already getting dehydrated. The sensation of thirst only appears when the levels of water in our bodies are already below normal. That's why we must drink water, even though we're not thirsty.

CARBOHYDRATES

Carbohydrates is a class of nutrients whose principle function is to provide energy to the cells in our bodies so they can do their jobs.

Through digestion, carbohydrates are broken down into smaller and smaller particles, until eventually they become glucose. Glucose is a type of sugar that is the primary source of energy for cells. There are two types of carbohydrates: simple and complex, depending on how long it takes our bodies to break them down into glucose. The difference between the two is especially important for children who have insulin resistance or diabetes.

To better understand simple versus complex carbohydrates, imagine little segments of glucose connected together, as if they were beads in a necklace. The longer the necklace, the longer it takes the body to separate the beads through digestion. That means it takes longer for the glucose to be broken down into individual units that cells can absorb for energy. With a short chain of glucose, it takes less time for the pieces to come apart and for the cells to soak them up as energy.

Simple Carbohydrates
Simple carbohydrates are made up of one or two units (beads) of glucose. They can also be made of other types of sugars that are similar to glucose, such as fructose, which is found in fruits, or lactose, which is found in milk. Fructose and lactose are quickly converted into glucose. Because they're "necklaces" with only a few beads, our bodies can break them apart quickly. That means glucose can be in the bloodstream within a matter of minutes. But in order for the sugar not to be left circulating in the bloodstream, the pancreas also has to work hard to produce enough insulin so the cells can absorb all that energy. When we eat a large amount of simple carbohydrates in one sitting (a large bowl of ice cream or a chunky piece of cake), the pancreas is forced to produce a whole lot more insulin to reduce the level of sugar in the bloodstream right away.

For people who don't have any trouble producing insulin, this isn't a big deal. But many Latino children suffer from insulin resistance. That means these children already have to produce a higher amount of insulin just to deal with the glucose that enters the bloodstream through a normal diet. When insulin-resistant children overload their bloodstreams with glucose, that's even worse for their insulin-producing cells. And remember that glucose that isn't burned off in a few hours is stored as fat.

The following are considered simple carbohydrates:

- *Sugars*, such as white sugar used to sweeten drinks or sodas or to make desserts and candy. White sugar is nearly pure glucose and doesn't have any fiber, vitamins, or minerals. Brown sugar and honey are also simple carbohydrates.

- *Refined flours*, an example of which is white flour used to make white bread, pasta, or desserts. Flours come from grains, which are complex carbohydrates, but artificially refining them with heat and other methods breaks apart the longer chains and allows the body to quickly covert them to glucose. During the refining process, flours lose much of their fiber, vitamins, and minerals. Sometimes manufacturers will add vitamins and minerals back to the flour after it's been refined.

- *Fruits* are also quickly converted into glucose, but the difference is that they contain fiber, vitamins, and minerals, which are essential for the healthy growth and development of children.

- *Milk* is a simple carbohydrate, but as with fruits, it contains vitamins and minerals that are great for a child's body.

Complex Carbohydrates

These are formed by long chains of glucose; the body takes longer to break these down. Because the longer chains of glucose take longer to get into the bloodstream, the pancreas doesn't have to make such a big effort to produce a huge amount of insulin to deal with a flood of glucose as it does with simple carbohydrates. When we eat complex carbohydrates, the pancreas produces insulin in smaller amounts over a longer time period. There are several types of complex carbohydrates:

- *Fibrous vegetables*: All vegetables contain fiber, but some more than others; for example, artichokes, asparagus, carrots, spinach, broccoli, romaine lettuce, and zucchini are excellent sources of fiber. Fiber is made up of glucose chains so long that our bodies can't digest them because we don't produce the enzyme capable of breaking them apart. That's why fiber leaves our bodies pretty much the same way it goes in. Fiber is an essential part of a healthy diet, because it helps move food through the digestive system, including the intestines. Also, fibrous carbohydrates take longer to digest, which means the glucose enters the bloodstream more slowly. In addition to fiber, complex carbohydrates also contain vitamins and minerals that are critical to a healthy body and the proper development of children.

- *Starchy vegetables*: Starches are the reserves some plants keep on hand to use during the germination process, before growing roots. Starches are also links of glucose our bodies can break down. But because they're long, we need more time to break them apart. Again, that means the glucose enters the bloodstream at a slower pace, making the job of the insulin that much easier. Pumpkin, jicama, potato, and sweet potato or yam are examples of starchy vegetables. These vegetables also contain fiber, and as with all vegetables, they do provide plenty of vitamins and minerals that help children grow.

- *Grains*: Grains are seeds that, just like starchy vegetables, contain a reserve of energy that provides them nourishment during germination. They are formed by long chains of glucose that our bodies break down slowly. Also, most whole grains are high in fiber, more than some vegetables. Some examples of grains include brown rice, corn, whole wheat, and oats. Grains contain many nutrients and essential vitamins that are important for growth. When some grains, such as wheat, are artificially refined and converted into white flour, they lose their nutritional benefits and are converted into simple carbohydrates. Even though some refined grains are enriched with vitamins, it's always good to combine them with whole-grain products.

PROTEINS

Proteins are found in foods like meat, fish, soy, milk, cheese, and eggs. Proteins are an essential part of our bodies that we need to regenerate constantly.

Inside our bodies, proteins act like little tools that allow us to do many different functions. For example, insulin, which allows glucose to enter cells, is a protein. Another protein is called hemoglobin, which transports the oxygen we breathe through the bloodstream to our cells. Other proteins act like bricks; they're the building blocks of our bodies. Fingernails and hair are made of a protein called *keratin*; many of the tissues in our bodies are made of *collagen*, another protein. As you can see, proteins are essential to proper body function, growth, and maintenance.

Elements called amino acids link themselves together to form proteins. Each protein has its own unique number and order of amino acids. To better understand how this works, think of the twenty-six letters of the alphabet. Every word you read in this book has a set number of letters in a specific order. But imagine if some words lacked letters or the order were changed around; you wouldn't understand what you were trying to read. The same thing happens with the amino acids that form proteins: If there aren't enough amino acids or they're not in the right order, the protein doesn't "make sense." It's like a poorly made brick foundation on a house that can't do its job supporting the structure. A balanced diet gives us the amino acids that proteins need to do the right job in our bodies.

Our bodies can actually make many of the amino acids found in proteins. But some, called essential amino acids, are only found in foods that have them. When we digest proteins they're broken down into amino acids and our bodies use them to create our own proteins, with their own set number and order of amino acids. But if we don't eat the foods that contain the amino acids we need, our bodies can't make certain proteins, thus causing some serious illnesses. Also, we must eat a sufficient amount of those amino acids to make sure our bodies have enough to create proteins. However, if we eat too much protein, the body will turn the leftover amount into fat.

Just like the rest of the cells in our bodies, proteins die after a certain amount of time (some after minutes, some after months). When these cells die they must be replaced. Children not only need to replace the cells that die, they also need additional proteins to keep growing. When children grow, their bones get longer and muscles and other tissues expand. All these parts need protein. That's why a balanced diet that contains all the essential amino acids is so important for proper growth and development of your child.

For babies who aren't able to eat adult foods, the ideal nourishment is breast milk, which contains every single one of the essential amino acids needed for growth. Mother's milk is a food that's tailored to a baby's every need. The amount of protein children need depends on how old they are. In later chapters, you'll find examples of what children of different ages need.

Sometimes it's difficult to understand exactly how much protein is in a certain type of food; the labels can be confusing. The amount of protein a food has isn't the same as how much the food weighs. For example, 29 ounces (100 grams) of chicken contains 22.5 grams of protein. The 100 grams of chicken isn't pure protein. So when you see that a balanced diet for a baby requires 30 grams of protein, that does not mean 30 grams of steak. Instead, the number refers to the amount of protein contained in the food. Not all food labels will tell you how much protein is in the food, because not all foods are required to have a nutritional fact label.

From a nutritional point of view, proteins are divided into two groups: complete and incomplete.

■ *Complete proteins*: These contain all the essential amino acids. In general, proteins that come from animals are considered to be complete proteins: beef, pork, fowl (chicken, turkey, duck, etc.), fish, milk, cheese, and eggs.

■ *Incomplete proteins*: These lack one of the essential amino acids and usually come from vegetables: Grains (rice, wheat), legumes (beans, lentils), and nuts, among others. However, some of these incomplete proteins can be combined to provide all the essential proteins. For example, even though rice and beans are classified as carbohydrates, when they're eaten together they make a complete protein. The beans are a source of the essential amino acid the rice lacks, and the rice provides the essential amino acid the beans are missing.

Most complete proteins come from animals and, therefore, are usually much more fatty than proteins that come from vegetables. In the next chapter, you'll find a list of all the different sources for protein.

FATS

Fats are found in foods such as butter, lard, and oil. You can also find different amounts of fats in foods such as meat, fish, or whole milk.

Our bodies do need a certain amount of fat to work properly. Fats are made up of fatty acids, which carry out all kinds of functions in the body: forming cell membranes, and the compounds our body uses to regulate blood pressure, blood clotting, and our heartbeat. Just as with amino acids, some fatty acids are considered *essential*, and we can only get them from the foods we eat because our bodies can't manufacture them. Fish oil, wheat germ oil, and nuts and seeds such as hazelnuts, almonds, and pumpkin seeds are very rich in essential fatty acids. Moreover, out of all the vitamins we need, fat-soluble vitamins can only enter our bodies dissolved in fat, because that's the only place those vitamins can be kept. Fat is also the principal source of stored energy for our bodies.

There are different types of fats; some are better for us than others.

- *Saturated fats*: These fats are solid at room temperature or in the refrigerator. Most come from animals or animal products. Some examples of saturated fats include lard, butter, fat from meats, fat from whole milk, and coconut and palm oil. Saturated fats increase levels of bad cholesterol, which can block arteries and cause heart disease.

- *Trans fats*: These are also known as *trans fatty acids*. These are created artificially through a process called hydrogenation. It involves adding hydrogen to vegetable oils to make them solid and keep them from spoiling. Trans fats or hydrogenated fats are used in many commercial products such as crackers and cookies as well as in fried foods such as doughnuts and french fries. Just like saturated fats, trans fats raise the levels of bad cholesterol in the blood and can lead to heart disease. The less saturated fats and trans fat consumed, the better. The labels on prepared foods will show you the amount of trans fats they contain. The words *partially hydrogenated* and *shortening* also indicate that a product contains trans fats.

- *Cholesterol*: Technically cholesterol isn't a fat, but it's found in animal products such as lard, butter, eggs, and meats. Cholesterol is needed to make hormones that carry out vital functions in our bodies. Our bodies make the cholesterol we need. Eating foods that are high in cholesterol raises the level of bad cholesterol in the bloodstream. However, saturated fats and trans fats raise the level of cholesterol much higher than foods that contain cholesterol naturally.

- *Monounsaturated fats*: These fats stay liquid at room temperature, but they can become solid in the refrigerator. Monounsaturated fats raise the level of good cholesterol. Good cholesterol, or HDL, helps eliminate bad cholesterol, or LDL, that sticks to the walls of blood vessels. Monounsaturated fats are found in olive, canola, and peanut oils. Although they are considered "good" they should be consumed in small amounts because they contain a lot of calories. You will find the right amounts in the Latino food pyramid.

- *Polyunsaturated fats*: These fats stay liquid at room temperature as well as in the refrigerator. Just like monounsaturated fats, these raise the level of good cholesterol. However, recent studies have shown polyunsaturated fats can alter lipoproteins (which transport fats through the bloodstream), so it's a good idea not to abuse them, or use monounsaturated fats instead. Polyunsaturated fats are found in vegetable oils such as sunflower, corn, and soy. There is one type of polyunsaturated fat that is really good for your health: omega-3.

- *Omega-3 fatty acids*: These are a type of polyunsaturated fat that, among other things, helps to reduce the levels of plaque of cholesterol that line the walls of blood vessels, protect the heart from irregular beating, and reduce blood pressure. Omega-3 fatty acids are found in fish such as salmon, albacore tuna, mackerel, and herring, as well as in nuts and linseed oil.

- *Omega-6 fatty acids*: Just like omega-3, these polyunsaturated fats are good for your health. Our bodies convert omega-6 fatty acids into *prostaglandins*. Prostaglandins are compounds similar to the hormones that regulate tissue swelling, blood pressure, and other functions in the heart, intestines, and kidneys. Omega-6 fatty acids are found in grains, eggs, poultry, and in the majority of vegetable oils. Recent nutritional studies show omega-3 and omega-6 fatty acids are only beneficial when we eat a balanced amount of the two.

Many obese Latino children have high levels of cholesterol and triglycerides in their blood. Even though fat should be part of a balanced diet, it's important to know what types of fat your child should avoid, which ones are most healthy, and in what amounts they should be eaten.

Vitamins

When you were a child, surely you heard your mother or father tell you: "*Come tus vegetales,* Eat your vegetables, they're good for you," or "You should eat more fruit, it's healthy," or "Finish your meat, it'll help you grow." Of course, now we tell our own children the same things, and with good reason. These foods are good for us because they're full of vitamins. We only need small amounts of vitamins, but they help our bodies do so many important things, such as growing and developing and fighting off infections.

Vitamins carry out specific tasks in our bodies. For example, the orange juice we drink in the morning contains vitamin C, which helps protect our gums; the vitamin K found in spinach keeps us from bleeding to death every time we're hurt. Vitamins are important for all of us, but especially for children during their growth years. Not only do vitamins help them grow but a lack of vitamins can cause diseases whose aftereffects will stay with them for the rest of their lives.

When it comes to vitamins, more isn't necessarily better, however, and sometimes more is worse. Excessive amounts of vitamins (in pill form or herbs or home remedies) can cause problems for the body. For example, there's a home remedy your mother or grandmother may have used that contains so much vitamin A it's toxic if you're not careful. The remedy is *aceite de hígado de bacalao,* cod liver oil. Some home remedies like this one, or some herbs, may appear natural, but it's always better to talk to your pediatrician or dietician before giving your child anything; there may be side effects you're not aware of. Vitamin supplements are not a substitute for a healthy, balanced diet. There is no supplement that can fix poor nutrition. Eating a variety of foods provides the ideal mix of vitamins, minerals, and other nutrients.

The foods we eat generally contain small amounts of vitamins. That's why they're measured in milligrams (mg), micrograms (mcg), or in international units (IU). It's important to be familiar with these measurements because they are listed on food and vitamin labels. The dosage of vitamins health experts recommend that we take every day (both children and adults) is expressed in these units. The dosage is called the recommended daily allowance (RDA).

To give you an idea of just how small these doses are, one ounce (that looks like four dice put together) equals 28 grams and one gram equals 1,000 milligrams (mg). One milligram equals 1,000 micrograms. Micrograms are also shown using the symbol µg. International units (IU) are a unit of measurement scientists use because some vitamins can't be compared by their quantities. In other words, the same amount of vitamin can have a very different effect depending on which vitamin you're talking about. For instance 100 mg of vitamin A isn't the same as 100 mg of vitamin C. So international units (IU) focus on the potency of the vitamin rather than the amount of the vitamin; the same IU means equal potency, but may mean different physical quantities, depending on the vitamins being compared.

Most foods also contain small amounts of vitamins. For example, green leafy vegetables (radish, lettuce, watercress, etc.) and red vegetables (radish, pumpkins, peppers, etc.) contain many of the essential vitamins our bodies can't produce. That's why the more variety you include in your balanced diet, the more benefits your child will reap.

Some vitamins are dissolved in fat (liposoluble vitamins); that's why your diet should include an adequate amount of fat. Liposoluble vitamins are stored in the liver, but too much can be toxic. However, the truth is it's more common to find health problems because of vitamin deficiencies than excesses. Another group of vitamins are the hydrosoluble vitamins, which are dissolved in water. These vitamins aren't stored in great amounts in the body, so it's important to obtain them by regularly eating the right foods.

Certain vitamins are known by letters, because when they were first discovered, scientists thought of using the alphabet to name them. Later, scientists discovered new vitamins that were part of the original vitamin or that technically (because of their chemical structure) were not vitamins. However, they performed equally essential functions in the body, and that's why they were given different names.

LIPOSOLUBLE VITAMINS

Vitamin A

Vitamin A isn't a single substance but an entire family of substances. Among the elements grouped under the vitamin A umbrella are:

- *Retinol*: Our bodies make good use of this form of vitamin A, which is found in foods such as **liver, fatty fish**, and **eggs**.

- *Carotenes*: These also go by the name A provitamins, because our bodies later convert them into vitamin A. Among carotenes, beta-carotenes are most easily converted into vitamin A. Carotenes are found in dark-colored vegetables, and fruits such as **red peppers, paprika spinach, broccoli, carrots, peaches**, and **tomatoes**.

Why children need vitamin A

- Essential for bone growth

- Maintains good eyesight; eyes can dry out without vitamin A

- Helps cells decide what they're going to be (a kidney cell or a skin cell) and to divide themselves

- Helps skin and mucous membranes stay intact, by preventing bacteria and viruses from entering our bodies

- Helps regulate the immune system, which fights off infections

Problems caused by a lack of vitamin A

Cases of extreme vitamin A deficiency are rare in the United States, even though they do exist in other countries. However, there are frequent cases in this country where minor vitamin A deficiencies occur because of a poor diet. Some of the symptoms of children who lack the proper amount of vitamin A include:

- Slow-developing bones and retarded growth in general

- Night blindness, or xerophthalmia

- Respiratory infections and diarrhea

- Poor defenses against infections

Vitamin D

Vitamin D is found in some of the foods we eat, and our skin can make it too when it's exposed to the sun or ultraviolet light rays. Vitamin D is commonly known as the sun vitamin. This vitamin is also found in **salmon, mackerel,** or **canned tuna,** although not in great amounts. The most common sources of vitamin D are foods that have been fortified with it, such as **vitamin D–fortified milk.**

Why children need vitamin D

- The main function of vitamin D is to maintain calcium levels in the blood (which helps bones to grow properly and keeps them strong) as well as proper levels of phosphorous (which helps to maintain bones, teeth, and other tissues).

- Recent studies have shown that vitamin D also helps to boost the immune system.

Problems caused by a lack of vitamin D

Small children are especially susceptible to a lack of vitamin D because their skeletons are growing rapidly. When they don't have a sufficient amount of vitamin D, they may develop rickets. Children with this disease suffer from poorly developed bones. Rickets was common in the last century, up until the U.S. government started a program that required milk to be fortified with vitamin D. Now rickets has just about disappeared. To ensure that your child has the proper amount of vitamin D, you should:

- give your child the right amount of milk to drink every day (you'll find the quantities appropriate for your child's age in the menus). If your child suffers from lactose intolerance (as many Latino children do), ask your pediatrician or dietician what other options you have for getting vitamin D; and

- make sure your child gets twenty to forty minutes of sun on the face and arms three times a week.

Our skin can't make vitamin D without ultraviolet light rays. But keep in mind, these rays can also damage and burn the skin. After about ten minutes, put sunscreen on your child. Once the sunscreen has been applied, the skin doesn't produce any more vitamin D because the ultraviolet light rays are no longer passing through. Regarding babies, the Academy of American Pediatrics recommends keeping them out of the sun. On the other hand, babies who are breastfed usually end up with a vitamin D deficiency; that's why your obstetrician may give you a vitamin D supplement to help make sure your baby gets enough.

Vitamin E
There are various types of vitamin E, but the one that's best absorbed by the body is known as alpha-tocopherol. Vitamin E is found in vegetable oils, especially wheat germ oil, and in nuts and seeds such as **almonds, sunflower seeds**, and **peanuts**, as well as in fruits and vegetables such as **broccoli, spinach, kiwi,** and **mango.**

Why children need vitamin E

Vitamin E's main function is to protect us against compounds called free radicals. Free radicals are strange elements that form in our bodies as a consequence of the chemical reactions that take place in order to obtain energy—and also when we come in contact with contaminants such as cigarette smoke or pollution. Free radicals damage cells and eventually destroy them; vitamin E reduces or prevents the damage.

Problems caused by a lack of vitamin E

Vitamin E deficiency is rare in humans, but when it does happen, because of a genetic abnormality or because of poor absorption, it can cause nerve degeneration in the hands and feet, anemia, and stunted growth.

Vitamin K

Vitamin K is essential for blood clotting. It's found in green leafy vegetables (broccoli, spinach) and in cabbage, cauliflower, and soy oil.

Why children need vitamin K

- Stops bleeding by clotting the blood during an injury

- Attaches calcium in the bones so they can grow

Problems caused by a lack of vitamin K

- Excessive bleeding and bruising

- Difficulty with blood clotting and anemia

- Stunted growth

HYDROSOLUBLE VITAMINS

Vitamin C

Vitamin C, also known as ascorbic acid, is only available to us through certain foods; our bodies can't make it. In the old days, sailors used to get deathly ill during long trips because they couldn't eat fruits and vegetables for months on end. *Guayaba*/**guava** is one of the foods that contains the highest amounts of vitamin C, followed by **strawberries, kiwis, oranges, lemons,** and **grapefruit. Green peppers** and **broccoli** are also rich in vitamin C.

Vitamin C isn't stored in our bodies, so it's necessary to consume some every day.

Why children need vitamin C

- Helps to create collagen, which is like the glue that holds our bodies together

- Protects cells from damage by free radicals

- Helps to absorb iron, critical to preventing anemia

Problems caused by a lack of vitamin C

- Scurvy, a disease that sailors of old times suffered from; muscles cramp, gums get inflamed, and teeth fall out

- Muscle weakness

- Less resistance to infections

Thiamin

This is also known as vitamin B_1. Our cells are unable to convert the food we eat into energy without thiamin. This vitamin is found in **pork, fortified breads,** and **whole grains,** as well as in **sunflower seeds, beans,** and **peas.**

Why children need thiamin

- Promotes growth

- Essential for healthy heart, muscles, and nervous system

Problems caused by a lack of thiamin

Beriberi, a disease caused by serious thiamin deficiency, can damage the heart and nervous system. In small children, beriberi can be grave.

Riboflavin

Riboflavin, or vitamin B_2, plays an important role in how our cells convert food into energy. Riboflavin is found in **milk, cheese, fried meats, green leafy vegetables,** and **nuts.** There are many **breads** and **grains** that are fortified with riboflavin. Light destroys this vitamin, so it's a good idea not to leave these foods in clear containers exposed to sunlight.

Why children need riboflavin

- Necessary for growth

- Maintains healthy skin, nails, hair, and mucous membranes (inside the mouth)

- Helps in the formation of red blood cells, which distribute oxygen throughout our bodies

Problems caused by a lack of riboflavin

- Stunted growth

- Swelling inside of the mouth and lips and a deterioration of the skin

Niacin

Niacin is also known as vitamin B_3. This vitamin plays a role in how all our cells obtain energy. It's found in foods such as **milk, cheese, poultry, fish, eggs,** and **lean meats.** Some **breads** and **grains** are fortified with niacin.

Why children need niacin

- Absolutely necessary for the health of the brain and nervous system

- Helps maintain the digestive system and skin

Problems caused by a lack of niacin

- A grave lack of niacin causes pellagra, a disease that leaves the skin and mouth covered in flaky sores

- A condition known as the three Ds: dermatitis, diarrhea, and dementia

Pantotenic Acid

This is also known as vitamin B_5. This vitamin helps convert the fats and sugars we eat into energy and it also helps our bodies create cholesterol. Remember, our bodies need cholesterol for proper brain function. Pantotenic acid is found in many foods. However, in frozen and processed foods, it often is lost. You will consume this vitamin by eating **eggs, fish, milk** and its derivatives, and **whole grains,** as well as **broccoli** and **cabbage.**

Why children need pantothenic acid

- Helps children grow by promoting the formation of new cells

- Necessary for the formation of antibodies, which help us fight off infections

- Helps to heal wounds

Problems caused by a lack of pantothenic acid

- Creates a greater sensitivity to insulin

- Muscle weakness, fatigue, and depression

- Stomach ulcers

Biotin

This vitamin plays an important role in the use and storage of the fatty acids that make up fats. Our own intestines can make biotin, but it's also found in many of the foods we eat. Some of the foods richest in biotin include **kidneys, egg yolks, brewer's yeast,** and **tomatoes.**

Why children need biotin
- Helps to process fats and certain amino acids

- Alleviates muscle pain and some skin problems

Problems caused by a lack of biotin
- It's rare, but a lack of biotin during the ages when children grow most can cause neurological abnormalities, weight loss, and hair loss, among other problems

- Raw egg whites keep biotin from being absorbed by the intestine

Pyridoxine
Also known as vitamin B_6, one of its principle functions is to help convert certain proteins into others by breaking them down into amino acids. This vitamin is found in foods such as **beans, lentils, garbanzos, nuts, eggs, meats, and fish.**

Why children need pyridoxine
- Essential for growth because it helps the body process the nutrients in many of the foods we eat

- Helps to make red blood cells

- Supports a healthy immune system

Problems caused by a lack of pyridoxine
- Nervousness, insomnia, loss of appetite, and weakness

- Lesions in the mouth, lips, and tongue

Folic Acid
Folic acid also goes by the name vitamin B_9. This vitamin helps our bodies create our own genetic code, which are the instructions that tell cells what organs they should form. It's found in most green leafy veg-

etables (**spinach, asparagus, broccoli**), **whole grains, legumes, lean beef, and fowl.**

Why children need folate or folic acid
- Important during the growth years because it plays a role in creating the genetic code that produces new cells in new tissues

- Works with vitamins B_{12} and C to help the body digest and use the proteins in the foods we eat

- Helps to create red blood cells

Problems caused by a lack of folate or folic acid
- Developmental abnormalities

- Poor absorption of nutrients as well as anemia

Vitamin B_{12}
The other name for this vitamin is cobalamin, but it's better known as vitamin B_{12}. This vitamin makes sure every cell in the body does its job correctly. It helps in the formation of red blood cells and myelin (a fatty substance that separates and protects nerves). Vitamin B_{12} is found in foods derived from animals, such as **liver, shellfish, meats, eggs, fish oil,** and **milk.**

Why children need vitamin B_{12}
- Improves concentration and memory

- Helps to regenerate bone marrow and red blood cells

- Helps the nervous system work properly

Problems caused by a lack of vitamin B_{12}
- Anemia and swollen tongue

- Nervous system problems

Minerals

Just like vitamins, minerals are chemical elements that our bodies just can't do without. Minerals can do great things: help our bones grow, help muscles contract, and send signals from the brain to nerves all over the body. There's more; minerals also keep all the fluids in our bodies in balance, including our blood.

Our bodies require some minerals in high concentrations; they're called macrominerals. Others called microminerals are only needed in small amounts. The interesting thing is, many minerals are toxic in high quantities and can cause serious illnesses in both children and adults. You should talk to your doctor before giving your child any type of mineral supplement.

MACROMINERALS

Sodium

The main function of sodium, along with potassium, is to maintain the liquids in our bodies in balance. For example, sodium determines the amount of water inside and outside our cells. This mineral also plays an important role in regulating blood pressure.

Nearly all foods have some form of sodium, especially salt. Some products have sodium added as part of the manufacturing process. Sausages, pickles, salted meats and fish, canned foods, salsas, snacks, and bouillon cubes all have a lot of sodium.

Sodium deficiency is rare. What's common are illnesses caused by too much sodium, such as high blood pressure, heart problems, or fluid retention. Some people take diuretics (products that help the body rid itself of excess fluids), herbs, or other home remedies to lose weight. But using these products without a doctor's supervision is quite dangerous, because you're not only losing water, you're also getting rid of vital minerals that can't be replaced just by drinking more water afterward.

Potassium

This mineral is closely related to sodium; they both help to control and regulate the balance of water in the body. Muscles need potassium to contract, including the heart, which can't maintain a consistent rhythm without this mineral.

Fruits, fresh vegetables, nuts, and **dried fruits** are sources of potassium, as are **potatoes.**

When our bodies don't have enough potassium, they show it right away: muscle weakness, nausea, fatigue, and confusion are some signs of potassium deficiency.

Calcium

Bones, teeth, and other tissues are made of calcium. This mineral is essential to their growth and regeneration. Children must have adequate amounts of calcium so they can grow up. But in addition to strong bones and teeth, calcium also has other functions in the body. For example, calcium helps blood clot when you get cut or injured. It also plays a role in muscle contraction and in sending signals across the nervous system.

This mineral is mostly found in **milk** and **milk products,** as well as in **canned sardines** and **green leafy vegetables.** One interesting aspect of calcium is that boiling the foods that contain it or freezing them doesn't change the amount of calcium in the food. Loss does happen, however, with other minerals. Your body needs vitamin D in order to absorb the calcium you eat. Vitamin D comes from certain foods, and our bodies can also make it when we expose our skin to the sun. Outdoor exercise helps with calcium absorption.

A lack of calcium results in soft and malformed bones. Children who don't have enough calcium or vitamin D get rickets.

Phosphorous

Phosphorous helps cells to divide, so obviously it's an important factor of children's growth. And along with calcium, phosphorous makes for strong bones and teeth.

Meats, eggs, milk, milk products, and **nuts** are great sources of phosphorous.

Because this mineral is found in so many foods, it's rare to find someone who suffers a deficiency. Moreover, phosphorous is added to some products such as cola soft drinks. Nevertheless, the symptoms of phosphorous deficiency include feeling run-down, weakness, lack of appetite, and breathing problems.

Magnesium

This mineral helps muscles to relax after they've contracted. It also keeps bones, teeth, and cartilage in good shape, helps to transport oxygen throughout the body, and assists in the transmission of signals throughout the nervous system.

Cocoa is one of the best sources of magnesium, along with **nuts, whole grains**, and **green leafy vegetables**.

Magnesium deficiency is rare, because this mineral is found in so many foods. The symptoms include: restlessness, weakness, high blood pressure, and convulsions. The intestine absorbs magnesium after digestion, but when a child has diarrhea, this doesn't happen. The loss of minerals and other nutrients can cause serious health problems for children.

Sulfur

Sulfur is one of the three amino acids that make up proteins. Without this mineral, proteins wouldn't exist. Sulfur is also present in the proteins that make up skin, hair, and nails. That's what causes the terrible smell when hair burns.

Sulfur is found in **cheese, eggs, legumes, meats**, and **nuts**.

A lack of this mineral can cause stunted growth, because the body can't make the proteins necessary for normal development.

MICROMINERALS

Copper

Without copper, our bodies wouldn't be able to make hemoglobin, which performs the vital function of transporting oxygen to all the cells in our bodies. This micromineral also helps to maintain our bones and tendons.

Copper is found in mollusks, especially **oysters,** as well as **liver, kidneys,** and other **organ meats.**

Copper deficiency causes anemia and stunted growth, but these symptoms are rare. Sometimes people can be poisoned by having too much copper in their bodies, for instance after eating foods cooked in copper or brass pots that are not properly lined with aluminum or stainless steel. Too much copper can cause permanent liver damage.

Iodine

Mental and physical fitness depend on iodine. Also it helps keep nerve and muscle tissues functioning properly.

The best sources of iodine are foods that come from the sea: **fish, shellfish,** and **iodized salt.**

This micromineral is plentiful in the sea. Some people who live in places far from the sea may have too little iodine in their diets. When children don't get enough iodine, their physical and mental development is stunted and they suffer an illness called cretinism. Manufacturers add iodine to salt to prevent this illness.

Iron

Iron is another micromineral that helps hemoglobin transport oxygen. Hemoglobin takes the oxygen we breathe in through our lungs and carries it to each and every cell in our bodies.

Liver, lean meats, sardines, and **green leafy vegetables** are great sources of iron.

Anemia is caused by a lack of iron (iron deficiency anemia is the most common of all anemias). Other symptoms of iron deficiency include fatigue, depression, heart palpitations, and low resistance to infections. Because women lose blood during their menstrual period, they need an extra daily dose of iron.

Manganese

Manganese helps build strong bones and muscles. It also plays a key role in insulin secretion and helps the body to carry out the myriad of complex chemical reactions that keep it functioning.

This micromineral is found in **nuts, whole-grain cereals**, and **green leafy vegetables**. Manganese deficiency is rare, but can result in poor bone development and lower glucose tolerance.

Chromium

This micromineral is needed so insulin will get glucose into cells. It also reduces high cholesterol levels. It's an important mineral for Latino children since they often have problems with proper insulin function and with high cholesterol.

Brewer's yeast (which you can find in most health food stores) is one of the best sources of chromium, as well as **liver, peas, American cheese, eggs**, and **whole grain cereal**.

A lack of chromium often results in symptoms similar to diabetes, such as weight loss and lack of insulin.

Cobalt

Cobalt is an essential part of vitamin B_{12}, which is in charge of making red blood cells and the protective layer that covers our nerves, called myelin.

Wherever you find vitamin B_{12} you'll also find cobalt, in foods like **liver, mollusks, meats, eggs, fish oil**, and **milk**.

By the same token, a lack of vitamin B_{12} also means a lack of cobalt, which results in stunted growth, anemia, and problems with the nervous system.

Zinc

This micromineral plays a role in the creation of insulin and translating the genetic code (the instructions) to make cells. It also gives the immune system a boost in fighting bacterial infections.

Fish, meats, legumes, and **whole-grain cereals** are the principle sources of zinc.

Insufficient zinc in the diet causes stunted growth, skin problems, hair loss, and keeps wounds from healing quickly.

Selenium

Selenium has many of the same characteristics as vitamin E; it protects us against free radicals, the compounds that make our cells get old. This micromineral also helps to prevent heart disease and stimulates the immune system.

Selenium is found in **fish, mollusks, meats, vegetables,** and **whole grains.**

A lack of this micromineral can cause stunted growth and even serious heart problems.

4

The Latino Diet

What's on the menu at your house? Latino, Tex-Mex, American food, or a mix of all three? This is the first question I ask my clients in my practice. Generally, Latino parents who were born in the United States have distanced themselves from the Latino diet, at least more than parents who were born in Latin America and emigrated to the United States as adults. The change away from a traditional Latino diet toward more American foods is usually not that healthy. The Latino diet, or the traditional foods in our native countries, is healthier in general than the typical Americanized diet. Here's why:

- The Latino diet includes more fruits and natural juices.

- Foods in the Latino diet are high in fiber (beans, vegetable soups, mangos, bananas), phosphorous (liver, meats, chicken, lentils, black beans), and niacin (pork, fish, meats, chicken, enriched white rice). All these nutrients are vital for the growth and development of our children.

- The Latino diet uses more complex carbohydrates, such as potatoes, legumes, rice, yams, and, especially, corn tortillas.

Corn (such as corn tortillas) is one of the most basic ingredients in the Latin/Mexican diet and it has many benefits for your children. Corn:

- Has no saturated fats or cholesterol and therefore is healthy for your heart.

- Is low in sodium and may help to keep high blood pressure down.

- Is a very good source of fiber that helps your digestive system and could balance your blood sugar levels.

- Is a good source of vitamin C, folate, thiamine, potassium, and iron.

But that isn't to say the Latino diet is perfect. There are two things that could use some improvement: The diet should include more dairy, such as milk (and the milk should be skim, not whole, which has more fat), and it should include more green leafy vegetables.

Among Hispanics the consumption of milk or dairy products decreases as we age. The myth among us is that only babies and infants need milk, and as children grow up, they can go to more "adult beverages" such as sodas and high-caffeine drinks. However, several studies suggest that dairy products not only are essential for the growth and development of children but may also help to control weight. In fact, there is evidence that dairy foods can keep adolescents from gaining excessive weight. Also, in the last few years, when the rates of childhood obesity have increased so much, children have been drinking many more sweetened soft drinks and consuming less milk.

Nevertheless, the traditional Latino diet is certainly a good, healthy starting point for both children and adults.

During my initial interviews with clients, I usually discover they haven't really stayed too far from the traditional Latino diet. But what they have done is exchange healthy ingredients for not-so-healthy ones. For example, many Latino children have given up on traditional *aguas frescas* or fruit-flavored water made with natural fruit juices and instead begun drinking sodas or sugared soft drinks. Here's another example: Instead of using corn tortillas, which are complex carbohydrates, many families have switched to white flour tortillas, because of their shelf life and versatility. However, these are made with simple carbohydrates.

A good idea to stay close to the Latino diet is to shop at the *mercaditos*, or local Latino markets, where you will find many of the real Latino ingredients for your meals.

The differences between Latino and American diets go beyond ingredients. There's also the issue of portions. In the United States, restaurants are really competitive. One way to get more customers in through the front door is to offer more food for the dollar. You've heard of supersizing; just a few cents more and you get an extra fistful of french fries. Also, portions that may be normal for an adult could be excessive for children.

Finally, exercise is an important factor to balance what we eat with what we burn. Before computers and video games, children spent most of their afternoons playing outside. In days past, children also walked to the neighborhood school. Due to different circumstances, Latinos today are the ethnic group that gets the least exercise, in the United States. The combination of American dietary customs, lack of exercise, and a genetic predisposition toward obesity are some of the reasons our Latino children are suffering an overweight health crisis. Fortunately there are ways to correct this problem.

The Latino Food Pyramid

You've probably heard of the food guide pyramid. It's a triangle chart that organizes the foods and portions we should eat every day to maintain a balanced, healthy diet. Every five years, the U.S. government publishes updated nutritional guidelines that give the general population an idea of what to eat to stay healthy. Aside from these dietary guidelines the government also publishes a food pyramid that establishes the portions and amounts for a healthy diet. The last food pyramid was published in 2005.

Using the U.S. government's guidelines as a starting point, I've created a Latino food pyramid that takes into account our culture, the foods we eat, and how we eat them. The Latino food pyramid will help you to easily understand:

- Which foods your child should eat.

- How much food is an appropriate portion.

- Which foods we should eat more of.

The Latino food pyramid starts at the bottom, with exercise and water. Exercise and water are the foundation of good health. Solely eating the right foods isn't enough to maintain a healthy weight. Next up in importance from exercise and water are fruits and vegetables, which provide the nutrients, vitamins, and minerals needed for proper growth and development. The next step holds beans, grains, cereals, and starchy vegetables. Continuing upward, the next step is proteins, such as low-fat dairy products and lean meats. Then we have a selection of the "healthy fats"; and finally, at the top of the pyramid are sweets, saturated fats, and trans fats. This is the smallest step in the entire pyramid, which means we should eat these the least. Underneath each one of the foods in every step, you'll also see exactly which vitamins and minerals they provide your child. Within the pyramid give priority to the lower levels of foods, since we tend to have a poor diet when it comes to fresh fruits and vegetables. However, all groups are essential (with the exception of the tip of the pyramid) for a balanced nutrition. You can print the Latino food pyramid at the book's Web site: www.healthylatinochildren.com.

Some examples of foods for each food group for children older than six are:

Low-fat dairy products: 2% reduced-fat, 1% low-fat, or fat-free (skim) milk; yogurt; cheese; ice cream; pudding.

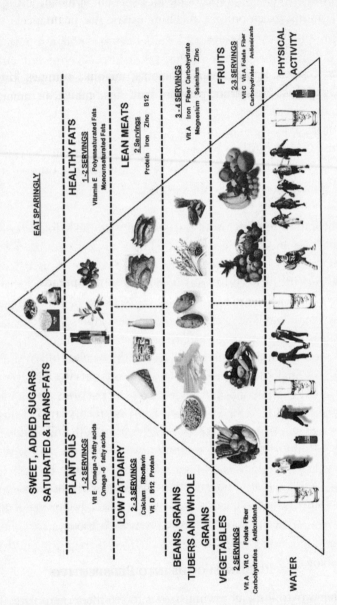

The Latino Food Pyramid

SWEET, ADDED SUGARS SATURATED & TRANS-FATS

EAT SPARINGLY

HEALTHY FATS
1-2 SERVINGS
Vitamin E Polyunsaturated Fats
Monounsaturated Fats

PLANT OILS
1-2 SERVINGS
Vit E Omega –3 fatty acids
Omega –6 fatty acids

LEAN MEATS
2 Servings
Protein Iron Zinc B12

LOW FAT DAIRY
2-3 SERVINGS
Calcium Riboflavin
Vit D B12 Protein

FRUITS
2-3 SERVINGS
Vit A Iron Fiber Carbohydrate
Magnesium Selenium Zinc
3 -4 SERVINGS
Vit A Vit A Folate Fiber
Carbohydrates Antioxidants

BEANS, GRAINS TUBERS AND WHOLE GRAINS

PHYSICAL ACTIVITY

VEGETABLES
2 SERVINGS
Vit A Vit C Folate Fiber
Carbohydrates Antioxidants

WATER

THE LATINO-HISPANIC FOOD GUIDE PYRAMID RECOMMENDATIONS ARE BASED ON 2400 CALORIES A DAY.
TO MAKE SURE YOUR CHILDREN OR ADOLESCENTS EAT WELL, REFER TO THE CHAPTER FOR THEIR AGE TO GET ALL THE NUTRIENTS AND CALORIES THEY NEED.

Vegetables: tomato, carrots, squash, broccoli, spinach, lettuce, cucumbers, onions, green onions, zucchini, asparagus, jicama, celery— green, yellow, and red vegetables.

Fruits: Grapes, apples, pears, bananas, melons, oranges, kiwis, mangoes, papayas, breadfruit, passion fruit, figs, guava, or tamarind. Any fresh or cooked fruit.

Grains: Corn tortillas, brown or white rice, potatoes, yucca, yams, taro, breads, cereals, pastas, noodles, lentils, beans, quinoa, amaranto, corn, plantains, bananas, and hominy.

Proteins: Lean meats including beef, pork, chicken, fish, eggs, tofu, shellfish.

Healthy fats: Olive oil, avocado, nuts, low-fat spreads, low-fat dressings.

Portions

Food quantities are measured in cups. The number of cups of food we need varies according to age. A portion is a serving size. Portions are the same for everybody, but the numbers of portions are different for a six-year-old child than for a twelve- or fourteen-year-old. In each one of the age-specific chapters in this book, you'll find which portions your child needs as well as sample menus. But as the saying goes, a picture is worth a thousand words, so along with the lists of foods that follow, you'll also find photographs that give you a better idea what exactly a cup of vegetables or grains looks like. Following is a list that gives you an idea of a portion size from each group.

PUTTING FOODS INTO PERSPECTIVE

Another way to look at serving sizes is to see them on a plate. The picture on page 75 is designed to show you how to choose foods from each of the groups of the Latino food pyramid (vegetables, fruits, grains, lean meats, low-fat dairy, and healthy fats) and benefit from a nutrient-rich diet. Let's see now how the Latino food pyramid is divided.

PHYSICAL ACTIVITY

Exercise is one of the most potent weapons we have in preventing obesity and helping your child lose weight. Because exercise is so important, the following chapters will explain what type of exercise is appropriate for your child's age. Physical activity or exercise isn't just about "going to the gym." Exercise may also be playing in the park, skating, riding a bicycle, or whatever activity you and your family find fun and interesting. Random exercise isn't enough. The key is to teach your children how to make exercise an enjoyable regular habit, something they can do for the rest of their lives. If children learn this lesson, they're much more likely to live long, healthy lives.

- Keep active: play outside, go to the park, help around the house, take the stairs instead of the elevator, take your dog or sibling for a walk, pick up your toys, walk to the store.

- Sports (done frequently) and/or recreational activities (done occasionally): basketball, soccer, kickball, skiing, volleyball, baseball, biking, swimming, jump rope, skateboard, running, dance, ballet, rowing, karate, etc.

WATER

Each individual needs a different amount of water depending on body size and composition, activity level, and the temperature and humidity of the environment. For a 2,000 calorie diet the body would need 2,000 to 3,000 milliliters of water (or eight to twelve cups of water) a day. Foods contribute about 1,000 milliliters of water (4 cups); therefore, the remaining four to eight cups of fluid should come from bever-

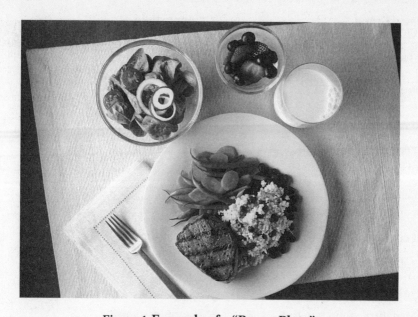

Figure 4: **Example of a "Power Plate"**

Photograph courtesy of the National Cattlemen's Beef Association

ages, preferably from water (see Appendix for water amount according to age).

FRUITS AND VEGETABLES

Fruits and vegetables are always part of a healthy diet, no matter our age. Children who are only months old start with cooked vegetable purées and fruit compotes. These foods provide key nutrients for growth and development. According to the Latino food pyramid, fruits and vegetables are the foods we should eat the most, throughout the day. Vegetable color is important: It's a good idea to eat green leafy vegetables as well as orange, yellow, and red vegetables, because they contain a lot of vitamins A and C, among others. Below you'll find a list of fruits and vegetables to include in your child's menu. Keep in mind that solid fruits have a lot of fiber, so they're more filling than

WHAT'S A SERVING SIZE, ANYWAY?

Food Group	Compare to
Vegetable	
1 cup fresh mixed veggies	1 fist or 1 baseball
Fruit	
1 cup of any fruit (i.e., sliced strawberries)	½ can beans (8 ounces)
1 small/medium apple or pear or orange	1 tennis ball
Grains	
1 cup whole grain rice	1 tennis ball
1 cup cooked spaghetti	½ grapefruit
2 slices of bread	2 CD cases
2 small tortillas	2 CDs
1 small/medium potato	1 computer mouse
2 small dinner rolls	2 soap bars
Dairy	
8 ounces/1 cup of milk	1 medium disposable cup
1 ounce/4 cheese cubes	4 dice
Lean Meat	
3 ounces (cooked) chicken breast or lean pork or red meat	deck of cards or cassette tape
3 ounces (cooked) grilled fish	1 checkbook
Healthy Fats	
1 ounce nuts	1 handful
1 ounce avocado	1 highlighter pen
2 tablespoons peanut butter	1 Ping-Pong ball

liquified ones. So it's always better to eat fruits as they are, instead of drinking fruit juices.

Vegetable Portions

One portion of vegetables equals:

1 cup raw vegetables
1 cup cooked vegetables

Note: Avoid choosing starchy vegetables (such as potatoes) within this category.

Orange, Red, and Yellow Vegetables:
- bell peppers
- carrots
- red peppers
- tomatoes, *jitomate, jitomatillo*
- salsa (tomato based)
- squash

Green Vegetables:
- asparagus
- broccoli
- Brussels sprouts
- celery
- cilantro
- chile peppers
- cucumbers
- dark green lettuce
- endives
- green peppers
- green beans
- green tomatoes
- *nopales*
- *quelites*
- spinach
- Swiss chard
- *verdolaga*
- watercress
- zucchini

Other Vegetables:

- artichokes
- beets
- cabbage, green or purple
- cauliflower
- *chayote*
- *chilacayote*
- eggplant
- garlic
- Jamaica flower
- mushrooms
- onion
- *poro*
- hearts of palm
- pumpkin flower
- soy sprouts
- Sprouts (alfalfa, clover, radish, etc.)
- turnip
- *xoconostle*
- *xonacate*

Note: Sprouts should be thoroughly cooked before eating them to destroy bacteria they tend to harbor. If you choose to eat them raw, buy them fresh, refrigerate them, and wash them with cold running water.

FRUIT SERVINGS

One serving of fruit equals:
  1 medium fresh fruit (or half of a big one)
  1 cup of cubed fresh fruit
  1 cup (8 ounces) of fruit juice (better to limit fruit juices to *one* a day)
  ½ cup of canned fruit
  ¼ cup of dried fruit

Note: Choose whole fruit over fruit juice.

Fruits:

- apple
- apple juice
- apricots, fresh or dried
- banana
- blackberries
- blueberries
- cherimoya fruit
- cherries

- *chico zapote*
- dates
- fresh pineapple
- grapes—green, purple, black, red
- grape juice
- grapefruit, fresh or juice
- *guanábana*
- guava/*guayaba*
- mango
- *mamey*
- mandarin orange
- *maracuyá*
- medlar
- melon—cantaloupe, etc.
- nectarine
- orange
- orange juice
- papaya
- passion fruit
- peach, fresh or dried
- *pitahaya*
- plums
- prunes
- raspberries
- raisins
- strawberries
- tamarind, pulp
- *tecojote*
- *tuna*
- watermelon
- *zapote*

BEANS; GRAINS, WHOLE GRAINS; AND STARCHY VEGETABLES

Within this category, you'll find several foods made from whole grains or refined grains. Whole grains include the outer "shell" of the grain (either it is not removed or it's added back after processing). These foods are absorbed by the body much more slowly than refined carbohydrates, which include processed foods and foods based on white flour.

GRAINS SERVINGS

A servings of grains equals:
    1 cup (example: 1 cup of *cooked* rice, dried beans, cereal, spaghetti)
    2 slices of bread
    2 small dinner rolls

2 small/medium tortillas

1 small/medium unit (example: 1 medium potato, yucca, malanga)

Beans and Grains:

The serving size for beans and grains is 1 cup (*cooked*); however, you can "mix and match" the grains by serving a ½ cup each of rice and beans.

- beans—1 cup
- chickpeas—1 cup
- lima beans—1 cup
- *gandules*—1 cup
- lentils—1 cup
- quinoa—1 cup
- rice (white, whole wheat, or wild)—1 cup
- pasta (whole wheat, white, or blended with vegetables)—1 cup
- noodles—1 cup

Cereals:

- breakfast cereal, low to moderate added sugar—1 cup or less
- cereal bar—1 unit
- Cheerios—1 cup or less
- cornflakes—1 cup or less
- granola (no fat)—½ cup
- muesli—½ cup
- oats—1 cup or less
- oat flakes—1 cup or less
- popped or puffed cereal—1 cup or less

Breads and Tortillas:

- *arepa*, plain—2 units regular size
- bagel—1 small medium size
- bread (white, whole wheat, pumpernickel, rye)—2 slices
- bread (French, Cuban, stick)—1 piece (4 inches long)
- buns for hot dogs or hamburgers—1 unit regular size

- English muffin—1 unit
- corn bread—1 unit (2 inches square, 3 oz.)
- corn tortilla—2 units small (6 to 8 inches across)
- croutons (low-fat)—4 tablespoons or less
- flour or whole-wheat tortillas—1 flour tortilla (6 to 8 inches across)
- *gordita*—1 plain small
- *jalapeño* bread—1 slice
- low-fat bread—2 slices
- pancake—2 units (4 inches across)
- *pupusas* (no filling)—1 unit small
- sweet bread (*media noche*)—1 regular unit
- taco shell—2 units (6 inches across)

Crackers:
- animal crackers—10 to 12 units
- crackers filled with cheese or peanut butter—3 units
- graham crackers—4 units (2½ inches square)
- melba toast—6 slices
- round appetizer crackers—6 to 8 units
- saltine crackers—6 to 8 small units
- whole-wheat crackers—4 units

Snacks:
- fig bars—2 small units
- plantain chips—12 small units
- popcorn (already popped), no fat—3 cups
- pretzels—1 ounce or one handful
- rice cakes—3 units (4 inches)
- tortilla chips—10 to 12 units

Starchy Vegetables:
- *camote*—1 small/medium size
- corn, yellow or white—¾ cup

- jicama—1 small/medium size
- malanga—1 small/medium size
- mashed potato—½ cup
- mixed vegetables (corn, peas, and other starchy vegetables)—¾ cup
- green peas—¾ cup
- potato, boiled or roasted—1 small/medium size
- pumpkin—1 unit (4 to 6 inches long)
- sweet potato—1 small/medium size
- yucca—1 small/medium size

DAIRY PRODUCTS

A serving of dairy products equals:

1 cup (8 ounces) (example: 1 cup of low-fat milk or low-fat yogurt)
1 to 2 ounces of natural or processed cheese
3 to 4 tablespoons of cheese (example: feta, Parmesan)

Milk and Yogurt:

- evaporated milk—½ cup
- nonfat or low-fat yogurt—8 ounces (1 cup)
- nonfat dry milk—¼ cup
- kefir, *jocoque*—½ cup
- skim or 1 percent milk—8 ounces (1 cup)
- soy milk—8 ounces (1 cup)
- whole milk—8 ounces (1 cup)
- yogurt, frozen, nonfat or low-fat—8 ounces (1 cup)
- yogurt with fruits, nonfat or low-fat—8 ounces (1 cup)

Less Fatty Cheeses:

- cottage cheese—2 ounces (4 tablespoons)
- cream cheese, low fat or nonfat—1½ ounces (3 tablespoons)
- feta, low fat or nonfat—2 ounces (4 tablespoons)
- *fresco* (fresh Mexican cheese)—1½ ounces (3 tablespoons)

- *de hoja*—1½ ounces (3 tablespoons)
- mozzarella—1½ ounces (3 tablespoons)
- Oaxaca—1½ ounces (3 tablespoons)
- *panela*—1½ ounces (3 tablespoons)
- Parmesan, low fat, grated—1½ ounces (3 tablespoons)
- white cheese (*queso blanco*)—1½ ounces (3 tablespoons)

Medium to High Fatty Cheeses:
- *asadero*—1 ounce
- American—1 ounce
- blue cheese—1 ounce
- Brie, Camembert—1 ounce
- cheddar—1 ounce
- Chihuahua—1 ounce
- *Cotija*—1 ounce
- Monterey Jack & jalapeño pepper—1 ounce
- provolone—1 ounce
- Swiss—1 ounce
- yellow cheese—1 ounce

MEATS, POULTRY, AND FISH

Meats, poultry, and fish are proteins. Some animal proteins can contain lots of fat, others are leaner.

One portion of meat or fish is equivalent to:
3 to 4 ounces of beef, chicken or pork, or veal
3 to 4 ounces of fish or shellfish

Less Fatty Meats and Fish:
- beef, lean
- bluefish (salmon, sardines, etc.)
- chicken without the skin
- lamb
- pork, lean

- ham, lean
- shellfish
- shrimp
- turkey without the skin
- white fish (tilapia, sole, hake, etc.)

Medium to High-Fat Meats:
- bacon—1 ounce (choose Canadian bacon)
- bologna—1 ounce (light)
- *carnitas*—1 ounce
- *machaca*—1 ounce
- *menudo*—1 ounce
- sausage, salami—1 ounce
- ham, regular fat—1 ounce
- turkey or chicken, with the skin—2 ounces
- sausage—1 ounce

Other Foods That Can Be Substituted for a Portion of Meats or Fish:
If you or someone in your family doesn't like to eat fish or meats, you can use the following foods as substitutes; however, the idea is that your child ends up liking all healthy foods, and you don't have to continue looking for "substitutes" even when he becomes a teenager. You'll find these alternate foods in different places in the Latino food pyramid. For example, beans are found in the grains category and cheeses are found in the milk category. But beans and cheeses also contain proteins.

- beans, lentils, etc. (grains)
- eggs (meat, fish)
- nuts, peanuts, almonds (healthy fats)
- low-fat cheeses (dairy)
- cottage cheese, low fat or nonfat (dairy)
- tofu (dairy)

- soybean (grain, vegetable)
- low-fat milk (dairy)

HEALTHY FATS

Your children also need fats in their diet, because these help them grow. Within the fats category, some are healthy, some aren't. Fats are more than just butter and oil. Fats are also found in cheese, dressings, or sour cream. Generally speaking, fats from plants are healthier than fats from animals. Nevertheless, fish oils are a great source of omega-3 amino acids, which are really good for us. Omega-6 amino acids are also good for us, and these are found in vegetable oils. Keep in mind the amount of fats you should eat every day includes not only the fats you use for cooking but also the fats you use in sauces and dressings to spice up your menus.

HEALTHY FAT PORTIONS

One portion of healthy fats is equivalent to:
- 1 ounce (example: 1 ounce of nuts, avocado, flax seeds)
- 2 tablespoons of peanut butter
- 1 spoonful of oil (example: 1 tablespoon of olive oil)
- 1 spoonful of spreads (example: soft margarine [free of trans fats], soft butter)

Healthy Fats:
- avocado oil—1 tablespoon
- corn oil—1 tablespoon
- guacamole/avocado—1 ounce
- dressing, Caesar, French or thousand island, low fat, nonfat—1 tablespoon
- mayonnaise, low fat, nonfat—1 tablespoon
- nuts (peanuts, almonds, pecans, walnuts, etc.) raw or roasted—1 ounce
- olive oil—1 tablespoon

- peanut butter—1 to 2 tablespoons
- soft margarine (free of trans fats)—1 tablespoon
- sour cream, nonfat—1 tablespoon
- sunflower oil—1 tablespoon

SWEETS, TRANS FATS, AND SATURATED FATS

Atop the Latino food pyramid, you'll find the foods you should only eat sparingly. Sweets rarely offer us vitamins or minerals, they make diabetes worse, and most contain unhealthy fats. Trans fats and saturated fats raise cholesterol levels. You should eat minimal portions of these foods because they contain a lot of sugar, saturated fats, and trans fats, all of which raise your cholesterol levels, and contribute to obesity. If you choose to offer these foods to your children, read the Nutrition Facts carefully for portion size and calories.

Desserts (*refer to the Nutrition Facts for serving size*):

- *até*
- brownie
- *buñuelo*
- *cajeta*
- *churro*
- cake
- chocolate chip cookies
- chocolate syrup
- cinnamon rolls
- coffee creamer
- condensed milk
- doughnut covered with sugar
- filled cookies, Oreo type
- flan
- fruit pie
- half-and-half cream
- ice cream with fat and sugars
- jams
- María cookies
- *palanqueta*
- *piloncillo*
- sweet bread

Saturated Fats and Trans Fats:
Saturated fats should be eaten in *limited* amounts. Our bodies don't really need a lot of saturated fats to work properly. On the other hand,

trans fats can be eliminated from our diets because they elevate the levels of cholesterol and the risk of heart disease. Starting in 2006, nutritional food labels now show how much trans fats are in a product. Some examples of trans fats include: margarine with hydrogenated oils, commercial fried products, industrial pastries, and potato chips. Avoid foods that have trans fats or where you see the words "partially hydrogenated" or "hydrogenated."

Saturated Fats (*1 tablespoon or less*):

- Alfredo sauce
- bacon
- blue cheese or ranch dressing, regular
- hollandaise sauce
- lard
- margarine
- sour cream, regular

Nutritional Food Labels: What Good Are They?

When obese children come to my practice with their families, one of the questions I ask the parents is if they use "nutritional food labels" when they go to the supermarket to help count calories and limit fat in the diet. Many say they try, but they're not really sure they know exactly what the labels mean. One of the goals I set for my patients is to learn how to use nutritional food labels, and to incorporate the information they provide into a healthy diet.

Food labels are the white squares (sometimes the background is a different color) on food packaging under the headline "Nutrition Facts." The information on these labels can really help you buy healthier foods for your family.

Grab a random can of food you've got in the pantry and follow along as we examine what the food labels tell us.

TYSON® CHICKEN BREAST STRIPS (BAGGED)

Nutrition Facts		
Serving Size 3 oz. (84 g) Serv. Per Container About 7		
Amount Per Serving		
Calories 120 Calories from Fat 30		
% Daily Value*		
Total Fat	3.5g	5%
Saturated Fat	1g	5%
Trans Fat	0g	
Polyunsaturated Fat	0.5g	
Monounsaturated Fat	1.5g	
Cholesterol	60mg	20%
Sodium	500mg	21%
Total Carbohydrate	1g	0%
Dietary Fiber	0g	0%
Sugars	0g	
Protein	21g	42%
Vitamin A		0%
Vitamin C		0%
Calcium		0%
Iron		0%
*Percent Daily Values are based on a 2,000 calorie diet.		

SERVING SIZE

Right under the label headline (Nutrition Facts) you'll find a line that reads Serving Size. In our example, the label reads Serving Size: 3 oz. (84 g). Or the serving size may be measured as the number of pieces of a product, such as 3 crackers; or measured by cups. That means the amount of calories, fats, cholesterol, sugars, sodium, and other ingredients shown on the label refers to that serving size, not the entire box, package, or bag.

SERVINGS PER CONTAINER

It's easy to overlook this important piece of information. In the example shown in the illustration, the entire package contains seven portions. This means if your child eats the entire bag of chicken strips, you'll have to multiply by seven all the nutritional information on the label. In other words, your child would have eaten seven servings' worth of fats, calories, sugars, etc. Again, the label tells you the nutritional content *per serving,* not for the entire container. Let's say you want to know the fat content of a specific food. A quick glance at the food label might make you think the fat content is pretty low. But to make sure, you should pay close attention to:

- The serving size: 3 ounces isn't the same as 6 or 9 ounces. It's not the same to eat one serving than 2 or 3 servings at once. And remember, the nutritional information refers only to the serving size, not the size of the container.

- The number of servings in the container: for example, the fat content on the nutritional label of a package of potato chips may not look like much at first. But if the fat content refers only to the amount of fat in eight chips and the package contains six servings, that means only eight chips contains the amount of fat you see on the label. And as we mentioned before, if you eat the entire bag, you've eaten six servings, and six times the amount of fat, calories, and sugars on the label.

CALORIES

Calories are a unit used to measure energy. The more calories a food has, the more energy it produces. The amount of energy we burn in our daily lives or exercising is also measured in calories. If we consume more calories than we burn, our bodies begin to store the extra calories as fat. Different people expend different amounts of calories in different ways. Children need fewer calories than adults, and really active people need more calories than sedentary people. For example, if your child eats two candy bars, each containing 250 calories, your child would have to swim about one hour or ride a bike for two hours to burn off these calories. As you can see, it takes a lot longer to burn calories than to eat them!

The calories that you see on the food nutrition label refer to the amount of energy per serving. In the example, one serving of chicken strips equals 120 calories.

CALORIES FROM FAT

Calories come from different sources: carbohydrates, proteins, and fats. A child who gets energy (calories) from sweets, sodas, and fatty fried foods is obviously not as healthy as the child who gets energy mostly from fruits, vegetables, and whole grains. In the case of the first child, fats and sweets will be the primary source of calories.

This part of the nutrition label in our example says out of the 120 calories in every serving, 30 will come from fat. Even though a child can gain weight by consuming too many calories regardless of where they come from (carbohydrates, proteins, or fats), the truth is, calories from fats are more likely to lead to obesity. It's important to keep in mind that fats are important for the development and growth of your child, but they have to be kept at a minimum. A healthy balance is needed because many times, calories from fats come disguised as other nutrients. This is why it's important to learn how to read and understand what's written on the food nutrition labels.

TOTAL FAT, CHOLESTEROL, SODIUM

Underneath the number of calories on a label you'll find the amount of fats, sodium (i.e., salt), carbohydrates, proteins, and other components in a particular food. Maintaining a healthy diet sometimes means reducing your consumption of some of the amounts that appear on this part of the label. For example, on the label shown on page 88, the total fats are 3.5 grams. Of the total fats, 1 gram comes from saturated fats, zero grams from trans fats, 0.5 grams from polyunsaturated fat, 1.5 from monounsaturated fat, and 0.5 grams from the ingredients.

In the column on the right, you'll see a list of percentages. These percentages refer to how much of a particular nutrient a person would consume, based on a diet of 2,000 calories per day, after eating a serving of the food in question. In our example, one serving will give us 5 percent of the recommended daily allowance of fat. One hundred percent is obviously the highest percentage of the % Daily Value, so after eating this food, we still have 95 percent or less to go before eating the maximum allowance of daily fat. If your child eats the entire package, it's the equivalent of seven portions, and 35 percent of the recommended daily allowance of fat. Reviewing the nutritional food labels will tell you whether your child is eating too much or not enough fat.

Trans fats don't have any recommended daily allowance percentage because there is no good amount of trans fats. They should be avoided completely. They raise the cholesterol levels in the blood and increase the risk of heart disease. Cholesterol and sodium are listed in milligrams, abbreviated as mg, and also in percentages.

TOTAL CARBOHYDRATES

These tell us that a serving of chicken strips (3 ounces) has 1 gram of carbs, or zero percent of the recommended daily value (based on a 2,000 calorie diet). Under the carbohydrates, as "subtitles," you will find "dietary fiber" and "sugars." This is for you to know how many calories from that gram of carbohydrates come from sugars and fiber. In this case, none of them do. The fiber percentage is there because we need fiber, and there is a lack of fiber in our diet. This figure will help you calculate the amount of fiber recommended daily.

PROTEINS

After the total carbohydrates listed on the label, you will find proteins. Usually, there is no percentage listed for proteins because in general we eat the right amounts. However, if your family eats meats that contain a lot of fat you should check the content and type of fats that protein or meat has. That's why, when you choose meat for your menu, the Nutrition Facts will tell you the type and amount of fats, but not necessarily the amount of protein. In this case, the amount of protein per serving is 21 grams, and 42 percent of the recommended daily allowance.

VITAMINS A AND C, CALCIUM, AND IRON

The last part of the food label tells you the amount of vitamins and minerals the food contains. These specific vitamins and minerals are listed on the label because these are the ones most commonly lacked by people living in the United States.

The percentage is the amount of vitamins A and C, calcium, and iron the food contains, in relation to how much one should eat every day. For example, if the food label says 15 percent calcium, your child still needs to eat other foods to get to 100 percent of the recommended daily allowance.

PERCENT OF DAILY VALUES

If there's enough space on the label, beneath the vitamins and minerals you'll find a paragraph that explains that these percentages are in relation to a daily diet of 2,000 calories. This information won't really mean much for your child, because each child has a different calorie requirement depending on age. For example, if your child needs less than 2,000 calories a day, the percentages he needs to eat will be less. This last paragraph is the same for all food labels.

If there is still more space beneath the recommended daily allowances for fats, cholesterol, sodium, and carbohydrates for a 2,000 calorie diet, you'll see another listing for the recommendations in a 2,500 calorie diet. And lastly, you'll see how many calories are in a gram of fat (9 calories), a gram of carbohydrates (4 calories), and a gram of protein (4 calories).

NET CARBS

On some product labels, you'll find the term *net carbs*. This term has become common thanks to the popularity of low-carb diets. Manufacturers of these products want to emphasize their low-carb content and this information is often prominently displayed on the front of the packaging. In addition to net carbs, you may also see this information described as effective carbs or net impact carbs.

There is no established government standard for net carbs, nor is there scientific agreement on exactly what it means. So depending on the product, net carbs could mean something different. What manufacturers are trying to show with the net carbs label is that their products offer fewer carbohydrates. To do that, manufacturers will substitute sugar with artificial sweeteners or sugar alcohols (natural compounds used as sweeteners). Many low-carb products are similar to products designed for diabetics.

But just because a product has a reduced amount of a certain nutrient doesn't mean it's low in calories. You'll have to watch the number of calories, even if the food is low carb or low fat.

INGREDIENTS

Generally the ingredients are listed on the back of the product. They are basically the ingredients of the "recipe," or everything the product contains. The ingredients present in bigger amounts are listed first and the ones with less amounts appear at the end. This is a very important list for people with food allergies.

The type and amount of ingredients will also give you an idea of how natural that product is. When grocery shopping, check the labels to see which products contain more natural versus artificial ingredients. Check for ingredients that we don't need for our nutrition, such as partially hydrogenated oils, also known as trans fats.

As you can see, food nutrition labels are full of information. You

don't really have to pace the aisles of the supermarket calculating percentages and grams. The most important things you should keep in
mind are: serving size and calories.

Still, it is useful to know the label can tell you exactly what you're
buying for your family. When you think about buying a box of cookies, a look at the labels will show you they're not all the same. The
amount of saturated fats and trans fats can vary greatly. The labels will
help you to choose the cookies with the least fat. The same goes for
buying a cereal with more fiber, or with less sugar. You can also see
which juice has the most vitamin C and whether it's been enriched
with calcium.

5

Nutrition During the First Months of Life

During my career as a pediatric nutritionist I've assisted pediatricians in many routine baby examinations. I remember a scene that played out almost every time, no matter which doctor's office I was in: A Latina mother would arrive with her baby—less than a year old usually; according to the measuring charts, the baby was overweight for its age and height. And even though the doctor dutifully warned the mother that the baby was overweight, she would break out in a huge smile.

There's no doubt that the growth your baby undergoes in the first months of life is essential to the proper overall development of the child. During the first year, children grow faster than they will for the rest of their lives. But growing healthily doesn't mean being overweight. Nevertheless, the majority of Latina mothers continue to believe a *gordito* or fat baby is a healthy one.

The idea of worrying about a baby's weight when it's only months old may seem extreme. And in fact, the real problem isn't that the baby is a little heavy during the first few months of life. What *is* important is that during these first few months the baby will learn attitudes and habits that later will be very difficult to change. If you've got a few *gordito* adults in your family, you know what I mean.

A child doesn't become obese from one day to the next. Children's obesity is a result of a combination of factors. The habits the child forms during infancy about nutrition, exercise, and what role healthy eating has in his or her family play an important part in whether a child will become obese. If *gorditos* make up most of your family, there's a big chance your child will be genetically predisposed to be obese as well. But being predisposed to obesity doesn't mean it has to happen. With the right attitude and armed with the right weapons, you have big chances to win the war against obesity.

Our culture sometimes has a good dose of *fatalismo*, a fatalistic attitude: "*Las cosas son como son*, things just are the way they are, and there's nothing we can do to change them." So it seems normal to think: "Son, if your grandfather and father were both *gorditos* you will be too so it doesn't matter what I do," or "*Dios así lo ha querido*, that's just the way things God wanted them to be." But when it comes to the nutrition of your child, you can lose the *fatalismo* attitude. In this chapter, we'll explain how to make sure your fears don't come true and we'll give you the knowledge and the tools you need to combat those genes your baby inherited. And if a doctor has already told you your baby is a little overweight, we'll tell you how to make things right.

As I said earlier, the first years of life are an important stage for your child, not only because of the physical growth but also because during this time frame you can establish the habits and limits on how your child will eat for the years to come. The later you begin to deal with the problem of obesity, the more difficult it is to correct it. The saying "*Más vale prevenir que curar*, an ounce of prevention is worth a pound of cure" is never truer than when dealing with obesity.

Infant Obesity Begins
During Pregnancy

The risks of having an obese baby, especially among Latina mothers, begin before birth. I am talking specifically about the last three months of pregnancy, when the baby begins to accumulate fat cells. The more fat accumulated during this time, the higher the risk of obesity.

Latino babies are at higher risk of accumulating a greater amount of fat cells during the last trimester because Latina mothers are three times more likely to be diabetic during pregnancy. This disease changes how insulin works in the mother. The result is that the baby receives much more "food" than normal through the placenta. In general, Latino babies weigh more than average at birth. Some studies have looked into whether this phenomenon is directly related to the higher rate of diabetes during pregnancy among Latina mothers. During prenatal visits, doctors can detect diabetes and can treat it fairly easily.

Nutrition is key to limiting the amount of fat your baby accumulates during the last trimester. The idea of "*comer por dos*, eating for two" has gone by the wayside. A mother only needs to increase her caloric intake by 300 calories a day to ensure that her baby is getting all the nutrients it needs (300 calories can equal a "regular" yogurt or a piece of bread and a glass of fruit juice).

Malnutrition can also affect the baby's development during pregnancy. When the mother's food intake isn't sufficient or healthy, the placenta might develop a greater nutrient absorption than normal. This too will influence the baby's weight at birth.

Nutrition During the First Months: Mother's Milk

You've probably already noticed the importance the medical community in the United States is beginning to place on breastfeeding. How often do you see a magazine article or television interview touting the benefits of mother's milk? Study after study has shown that the most appropriate nutrition for a newborn comes from its mother. Mother's milk has just the right amount of nutrients for a newborn to grow and develop healthily. There isn't a single formula on the market that reproduces the makeup of breast milk. Some of the scientifically proven benefits of mother's milk are that it:

- Protects the baby against gastrointestinal infections and diarrhea.
- Protects the baby against ear and respiratory infections.
- Helps in the neurological development of the baby.
- Protects the baby against allergies.

As if that weren't enough, the makeup of mother's milk changes as the baby's nutritional needs change. In the grocery store, you'll never find a formula designed for a baby that's three months one week old, or four and a half months old. But that's exactly what breast milk can do; it changes to meet the specific nutritional needs of your baby as he develops.

Breastfeeding is also beneficial for the mother. It helps control bleeding after delivery because it helps the uterus return to its normal size; breastfeeding also helps to ward off breast and ovarian cancer.

But besides all this, there's another good reason to breastfeed: Research shows that it helps control obesity in children. Just two months of breastfeeding can make a difference in whether your child will be obese. And the longer you breastfeed, the less likely it is your child will be overweight.

Latina Mothers and Breastfeeding

It's likely your grandmothers, aunts, or other female family members from past generations breastfed their babies, some with more success than others. In centuries past, there really wasn't an alternative. But during the 1940s, as more and more baby formulas came to market, many working women began to move away from breastfeeding their children. For example, in the United States during the 1940s, only one in four women chose to breastfeed. Among Latina mothers living in the U.S., breastfeeding was rare. However, during the 1960s, the tendency to avoid breastfeeding started to change as studies began to show the benefits of mother's milk.

During the last few years federal and state governments and other institutions have promoted breastfeeding through public service campaigns directed toward Latina mothers. And these campaigns have worked. In the past ten years, there's been a huge increase—48 percent—in the number of Latina women who've chosen to breastfeed. Today, seven of every ten Latina mothers breastfeed.

The American Pediatric Association and other experts recommend breastfeeding during the first year after birth. But the reality is, of the seven Latina mothers out of ten who do breastfeed, only three continue to do so after the baby reaches six months of age.

Latina mothers are heavily influenced in their decision to breastfeed or not by their husbands, partners, mothers, and other relatives. Latina mothers are likely to choose formula if the father doesn't like breastfeeding (for example, some men don't like the idea of their partners breastfeeding in public), or if their mothers had a bad experience with breastfeeding. We all know how much influence *la opinion de la familia*, the opinions of family members, have.

Even among Latina mothers who do have family support, few continue to breastfeed beyond six months. One of the most common reasons given for stopping breastfeeding is the perception that the baby isn't getting enough milk or that the milk isn't of good quality anymore and therefore the baby is not gaining weight as he or she should. This can be the beginning of obesity problems for many Latino children.

"My Baby Isn't Gaining Enough Weight."

During the first months me angustié mucho, *I was really nervous and worried. I thought Pedrito wasn't gaining all the weight he needed to. His legs seemed so skinny! My mother agreed, saying the baby must not have been getting enough to eat. When I squeezed my breasts, it didn't seem as though very much milk was coming out. That's when I began to use formula. At least that way, I knew for sure how much he was eating.*
—Leticia Pérez, twenty-nine

Leticia's baby, Pedrito, was the right weight according to his pediatrician. But like many Latina mothers, Leticia didn't believe it. She had the perception her baby was too thin, a perception that didn't correspond with reality.

When most Latina mothers fear their babies aren't getting enough to eat through breastfeeding, they begin to supplement the mother's milk with formula. A vicious cycle begins. On one hand the mother begins to produce less milk naturally, because the baby demands less breast milk. On the other, the baby is getting extra calories from the formula. Some Latina mothers will begin to feed the baby cereals and even some other solid foods before four or six months to help the baby gain weight (or to help him sleep longer). Scientific studies have shown that this practice can lead to asthma or other allergies in the future.

"I'm Not Making Enough Milk"

Another factor that can make mothers think their babies aren't getting enough to eat is that it's difficult to really know how much breast milk the baby is consuming. Unless you're using a breast pump, it is hard to know just how much food the baby is eating. However, mothers do know for sure when feeding formula from a bottle.

Mother's milk begins to appear two to three days after birth (sometimes longer if the birth was by cesarean). Many mothers worry that their babies aren't eating anything because they don't see milk flowing from their breasts. But even though you may not see it, your breasts are producing small amounts of a yellowish clear liquid called colostrum, just the right amount the baby needs during the first few days of life. Remember that the baby's digestive system is only beginning to work and it can only handle very small amounts of food at a time.

My recommendation is to trust your body and *la Madre Naturaleza*, Mother Nature. If there aren't any other illnesses or complications, you and your baby are adapting perfectly to each other's needs. It's normal for babies to lose a little weight after birth. But they're born with some energy reserves to help them make it through this initial transition period from the womb to the outside world.

Besides, there are ways to know if the baby is eating properly without having to measure your milk, as was proven by one study. The study monitored babies between two and three days old and weighed them on a sensitive electronic scale before they were breastfed. Then, all the signs indicating that the baby was eating were recorded (suction on the breast, swallowing noises, etc.). Finally, the babies were returned to the sensitive scales. In every case where there were signs that the baby was indeed feeding, the scales showed the babies had gained between 0.9 ounces and 1.3 ounces. So *esté tranquila*, rest assured, because even if you think you don't have enough milk, your baby is getting enough to eat if he or she:

- Latches well onto the nipple.
- Suckles.
- Makes swallowing noises.
- Dirties between one and four diapers a day with feces.
- Wets between five and six diapers a day with urine.

If you use a breast pump, don't compare your production with other mothers. Although you may have less milk, that doesn't mean you're not giving your baby all the nutrition he needs. If your pediatrician says your baby is growing and developing just fine, you don't have to worry.

"My Milk Isn't Any Good"

Latina mothers also worry about the "quality" of their breast milk. The truth is, all breast milk has the same ingredients no matter which woman is making it. All women, really. Even women who live in countries where they can't have balanced diets or where they don't get enough calcium—their milk has the same levels of calcium and other nutrients as women of other countries. Unless there's an illness or a medical problem, one mother doesn't make better milk than others. What does happen is that the composition of the milk is different depending upon and according to the stage of the baby's development. Within the same breastfeeding session, the makeup of the milk changes. In the Appendix, you'll find several telephone numbers of organiza tions that can answer your questions about the quantity and quality of your breast milk.

What has been proven to affect the amount of milk you produce is giving your baby formula when he really doesn't need it. The more formula you give your baby, the less the baby will eat from your breasts and, as a consequence, the less milk you will produce.

Now, I'm not saying breastfeeding is for everyone. There are some personal and medical circumstances that could make breastfeeding impossible. But under normal situations, you should relax and feel confident in your ability to breastfeed your baby.

Latino Myths About Breastfeeding

Our culture is rich in ancestral traditions and myths about, well, nearly everything. Breastfeeding is no exception, and it's normal for mothers, especially first-time mothers, to get all kinds of advice and tips from relatives and friends. Even though it's been scientifically demonstrated that many of these myths are not true, they can still create a lot of anxiety for mothers who are trying to figure out how to breastfeed. Some of the most common myths include:

- *Anger and distress can make the milk go bad or dry up.* Luckily, being angry and upset does not change the way mother's milk tastes. If the mother is really anxious about something, it's possible she might have to work a little harder to produce milk, but it certainly doesn't disappear altogether. As soon as the mother relaxes, her breasts will begin to produce milk again. In addition, breastfeeding your baby will help you to relax. A woman's body relaxes in a natural way when it's breastfeeding.

- *When the breast milk* se agua, *turns watery, you must stop breastfeeding.* This is one of the reasons many Latina mothers begin to give their babies formula as a supplement to breast milk.

At the beginning my milk had this rich white color, but after a few weeks I saw it was turning into a lighter and watery color. My aunt told me that my milk se estaba aguando, it was turning watery. I was afraid my baby was not getting enough nourishment.
                                        —*Ángela, twenty-three years old*

Breast milk doesn't always look the same. At first, the milk that's produced has less fat in it and that's why it looks a little different. And even during the same breastfeeding session, the milk can change appearance. The milk that comes out during the first few minutes has more water and sugar and less fat to satisfy the baby's thirst. Then the amount of fat begins to increase to make sure the baby gets all the nutrients he needs. Also, don't compare the color of breast milk with formula, because they look very different. The natural appearance of mother's milk is indeed more watery and clear than formula.

- *Mothers should eat cooked oats in milk or malt, fig leaves, or peanuts to produce more milk, and they should try to avoid "cold" foods.* There are no scientific studies that say you shouldn't eat these foods nor is there any problem with eating them while you are breastfeeding. Problems arise when mothers try to eat only the foods they think will help them produce more milk and avoid eating healthy, balanced diets. Breastfeeding mothers as well as pregnant women need to eat as healthily as possible because their bodies are working extra hard. Many Latino cultures still believe the body needs a balance between *el frío y el calor,* "cold" and "hot." The period after delivery is considered a "hot" stage where mothers should avoid "cold" foods. The danger in this practice is that some of those "cold" foods are actually healthy for the mother to eat while she's breastfeeding (or at any other time): fruits, vegetables, and others. On the other hand, eating too much while breastfeeding will not increase the amount of milk you produce, but it will increase the number of pounds you put on. What increases the production of milk is the act of breastfeeding; the more you breastfeed, the more milk you will produce.

- *Breastfeeding mothers shouldn't eat beans, jalapeños, or chocolate.* You can eat pretty much anything you want while breastfeeding. But if you think a certain food affects your baby, try avoiding it for a couple of days to see what happens. Some babies indeed are sensitive to the taste of breast milk when the mother has eaten garlic or cabbage. Finding out is simple: Eat one of the problem foods at a time and see what your baby does.

- *When the breasts become softer it means you're not producing enough milk.* After two or three weeks of breastfeeding, some mothers worry that their breasts aren't as full as they were right after delivery. They may not be, but that's fine. Sometimes the breasts of postpartum mothers (especially first-time mothers) become inflamed or swollen after delivery. As the days of breast-feeding go by, that inflammation disappears. The production of milk stays the same, only without the inflammation.

- *Mothers shouldn't let their babies eat the yellowish liquid that comes out of the breasts during the first few days after delivery.* Fortunately this myth isn't too widespread and many mothers know that this yellowish liquid, called colostrum, is the best feeding they can give to their babies. Colostrum is rich in easily absorbed proteins, minerals, vitamins, and other nutrients your baby's little body needs during the first few days after delivery. And that's not all: Colostrum is also transferring your antibodies to your baby to help him fight many of the same diseases you've been exposed to.

- *My mother didn't produce much breast milk so I won't either.* All women produce milk for their babies, unless they've got a specific medical problem with their breasts. It's more likely that your mother didn't have anyone to help her figure out just how to breastfeed her babies or what she could expect the first days after delivery.

My mother says that she couldn't breastfeed me because she didn't have enough milk. She had to give me formula instead. Now that I am breastfeeding my baby I wonder if the same will happen to me.
—Ana, thirty-two years old

Today, there are all kinds of consultants who can help you learn what to do, and how to do it successfully.

These are only a few of the many myths about breastfeeding. You probably know a few more yourself. Don't think your breast milk isn't good or isn't enough for your baby. Ask your pediatrician about it before supplementing your breast milk with formula. The best way to figure out if you're producing enough milk is to see how your baby grows. If the pediatrician says your baby is growing fine, then that means your breasts are working fine too.

Breastfeeding Difficulties

Just because breastfeeding is a natural process and just because doctors and specialists recommend it, that doesn't mean it's easy to do. Some mothers are successful right from the beginning, while others run into problems all along the way. Yes, breastfeeding is natural, but it requires some learning on the part of the mother and the baby as well.

I have breastfed all my children and so has Lourdes, coauthor of this book. And believe us, it was not easy, especially with our firstborns. However we knew that it was the best we could do for our children so we persevered. After the first weeks, when we were settled in a schedule, things were much easier. Not only was it worth it but we saved a lot of money. Breastfeeding can save you at least $1,500 a year.

In the olden days, when families all lived close together, there was always a grandmother, aunt, cousin, or sister who was willing and able to help the new mother figure out how to breastfeed. There were even wet nurses around who had breast milk available to share, if the mother was having trouble feeding her own children. Today mothers who don't have family around to help them through difficult breastfeeding times could feel very alone. The good news is that even if family isn't nearby, there are others who can help. In the Resource Guide at the end of the book, you'll find telephone numbers and addresses of experts who can help you with your breastfeeding problems for free. Even within your community you may find support groups for mothers who want to breastfeed. These meeting are usually quite useful, because in addition to providing some helpful tips, it's a place were you can share your struggles with breastfeeding with other mothers in the same situation, and that can be a great relief.

How Long Should I Breastfeed My Baby?

The American Pediatric Association recommends breastfeeding the baby until he's one year old so he will get all the benefits from mother's milk. As the months pass by, the baby's growth rate changes, as well as the times he needs to eat, both during the day and at night.

Each breastfeeding session can last from ten to twenty minutes on each breast. During the first few days and weeks, the baby probably needs to be fed every two to three hours (between seven and ten times a day and once or twice per night, maybe more). But as he grows and gets better at feeding, he will take less time to eat and can go for longer between feedings. It's normal for a mother to breastfeed every hour and a half to three hours; newborns eat little but often. Below you will find a chart with the approximate times you will be breastfeeding your baby as the months go by.

Months	Number of nursings per day
0–2	8–12 times or more
2–4	8–10 times or more
4–6	4–6 times or more
6–8	4–6 times
8–10	3–5 times
10–12	3–4 times
12 and up	1–3 times

Don't give your baby water if he's breastfeeding; the breast milk will be enough to keep your baby hydrated. However, you should talk to your pediatrician if you live in a place where it's really hot.

To make sure your baby is getting all the food he needs, check the number of diapers you change: one to four dirty diapers and five to six wet diapers every twenty-four hours means you're on track. During the first weeks, you shouldn't let your baby go for longer than four hours without feeding. Wake the baby up if he's asleep. Speak to the pediatrician if he is not waking up to eat.

All in all, breastfeeding is work and it requires effort and commitment on your part. For some mothers it comes easy, for others it's a pain. But remember it's a learning process and you'll improve the more you practice. The first few weeks in particular can be hard. Your nipples may hurt or burn. It's tedious to feed your baby at both breasts every few hours, and you'll probably feel tired. Still, if you can make it through this first stage, you'll find easier times are to come.

When Breastfeeding Is Not an Option

Even though a mother wants to breastfeed, sometimes this might not be possible. First of all, breastfeeding requires time and dedication. Some women have to return to work only a few weeks after giving birth and their workplaces don't offer the support they need to pump their breasts in a regular way in order to keep producing milk. Other times there are problems in the process of breastfeeding that could make it difficult for the mother to continue. Some of the most common difficulties are:

- Breast pain.
- Cracked or bleeding nipples.
- Breast infections.
- The baby has difficulty taking the nipple.
- The mother is too tired trying to nurse day and night.
- A prior breast surgery.

Medical treatment or the advice of a breastfeeding expert can help overcome some of these problems (see the Resource Guide for where to find help). But at times, in spite of all the efforts, breastfeeding just isn't possible.

> *I really tried, but it was just not possible. My nipples were bleeding, the baby didn't take the nipple right, and she was hungry all the time. She wanted to be nursed every hour and I was totally exhausted. When my breast got infected I really couldn't keep it up. I wanted so much to breast-feed her! I still feel bad about not being able to.*
>
> *—Guadalupe, thirty-six years old*

No se sienta culpable, don't feel guilty if you can't breastfeed or if you've decided you don't want to at all. You'll know when you've reached your limit, and a happy, well-rested mother is sometimes a better option than a breastfed baby. Even though mother's milk is better, there are many babies who have been raised and thrived on formula.

Types of Formula

You can find all kinds of formulas in the stores today: with or without iron, made of soy, without lactose, ready to serve in liquid form, in powder form, and even some with fatty acids that mimic those in breast milk.

Talk to your pediatrician about what type of formula is most appropriate for your baby. Generally, pediatricians will recommend formulas with iron, especially after the fourth month.

As far as the newer formulas with the fatty acids, docosahexaenoic and arachidonic (DHA and ARA) acid, they're usually more expensive than the regular ones. The companies that make these newer formulas insist they're better for brain development and eyesight. Mother's milk does contain these fatty acids. The amount depends upon what the mother eats. These fatty acids are found mainly in fish, red meats, and eggs. But there has yet to be a study published that firmly establishes whether these newer formulas will improve your baby's brain function or eyesight.

How Much Formula Should I Give My Baby?

Your pediatrician knows best just how much your baby should be eating, but to give you an idea, here's a chart describing what a baby should eat during the first twelve months.

Age	Amount	Feedings per 24 hours
1 week	2–3 ounces	7–10
1 month	2–4 ounces	6–8
2 months	5–6 ounces	5–6
3–5 months	6–7 ounces	5 6
6–8 months	6–8 ounces	4–5
8–10 months	4–5 ounces	4–5
10–12 months	6–8 ounces	3–4

Note: Formula-fed babies may need water; check with your pediatrician.

When babies go through growth spurts, they may want to eat more and more often. Generally, once the spurt is over the baby will return to its normal feeding schedule.

How to Tell If Your Baby Is Full

During the first days or weeks after delivery, it's hard for parents to tell if the baby is crying because of hunger, discomfort, or for some other reason. Too often it's easy to think the best thing to do is feed the baby to calm him. But even though at the beginning it's difficult to tell, you can learn when your baby is crying because he is hungry and when he is crying because he is uncomfortable, sleepy, or bored. And if you do, you've mastered one of the best tools in the fight against obesity. When you can distinguish the reasons your baby is crying, not only are you avoiding overfeeding but you are also teaching your baby that eating isn't the solution to every discomfort or spate of boredom he feels. Studies have shown that obese people have a difficult time figuring out whether they want to eat because they're hungry or because of something else, and they tend to eat as soon as something begins to bother them.

A healthy newborn knows when she's eaten enough and will begin to give signals that she doesn't want any more milk. Some of the signs to look for include:

- Letting go of the breast or bottle nipple.
- Pulling her head away from the breast or bottle.
- Closing her mouth.
- Arching her back.
- Showing interest in something else that doesn't have to do with feeding.

If your baby is getting formula, it's especially important to watch and learn to respect these signs when your baby starts to show them. With formula, you have more control over what your baby eats, not only because you can see just how much she eats by looking at the bottle but also because it's less likely the baby will reject the bottle. During breastfeeding, the baby is an active participant and has to suck hard to get the milk to come out; when the baby doesn't want to eat, it's very difficult to force her. But a bottle is different. Even though the baby has to do some sucking to get the milk to come out of the bottle, she has to work much less and sometimes all she has to do is swallow. So if you feed your baby from a bottle, make sure you watch for signs the baby's had enough. Remember, the size of her stomach during the first weeks is the size of a baby's fist and it could be full even before finishing a couple of ounces.

At the same time, it's important to learn the signs that your baby is hungry, so you can feed her when she asks and be able to know if she is complaining about something else. Some of the signals that a baby is hungry include:

- Opening the mouth and searching for a breast or bottle.
- Sucking randomly.
- Sucking the hand or fist.

Don't wait for the baby to cry from hunger. It's a good idea to set up a schedule, albeit a flexible, individualized one. If your baby is hungry before three hours pass from the last feeding, don't wait to feed her. Sometimes if you wait too long, the baby can get so upset it's difficult to get her calmed down enough to where she wants to eat again.

Breastfeeding is definitively a very important stage in developing the first healthy eating habits in your baby. Over the next few years, your child will learn to eat with your help. If you offer her proper foods as choices, allow your child to determine her own appetite, and establish a family atmosphere that supports physical activity, then you will be taking the first steps in preventing obesity and its consequences.

6

Nutrition from Breastfeeding to Two Years

The time from just less than one year up to two years of age is one of the most active learning phases of your child's life. From one year to two, children will speak their first words, take their first steps, and start to eat on their own. So the goal is to have children also learn some good eating habits during this time period, habits they can rely upon for the rest of their lives.

This time period will be trying for you, as you attempt to get your child to eat properly. Your child will be exploring and learning and still doesn't really know that a cup is for drinking. Expect milk to end up in hair and rice on the walls.

My first child, Carlos, was a pretty calm kid. But when his sister Carolina came along, the tranquility ended. When she was six months old, Carlos was twenty-one months. It was challenging to organize feeding two different babies of two different ages. When Carolina ate baby food, Carlos was by this point experimenting with "normal" food. Carolina had to be fed, Carlos tried to eat on his own. I had to use all my knowledge; I graduated as a dietitian at home as well as at the university. Lourdes, coauthor of this book, is a mother of four children. She also has vivid memories of her children's first meals, and how more food would end up everywhere except on their plates.

> I have a picture of Adriana that still makes me laugh. There was mashed sweet potato everywhere, in her hair, ears, nose . . . and even on the wall. But to be honest, I was not laughing that much then!
> —Lourdes, forty-two years old

Just about the time children give up their bibs, they often become finicky—they'll refuse to eat certain foods and always demand others. The key for you as a parent is patience. Your child isn't going to starve or have growth problems just because the plate isn't clean at the end of every dinner. On the other hand, children can learn some bad eating habits if parents begin to pressure too much. The best thing for parents to do is to look at the big picture: what your child is eating over the course of a week, instead of focusing on what's eaten at each meal. So be patient and have faith that this is a phase and that it will pass.

From Four to Six Months: Introducing Cereal

At four to six months, your baby is now ready to begin eating something new: cereals. The American Academy of Pediatrics recommends that breastfed babies satisfied with milk should not be given solids until six months of age. However, you should talk to your pediatrician if before that time your baby doesn't seem satisfied just with milk.

Remember that before four months your baby still isn't capable of digesting cereals or any other solid foods, so don't try. Always follow the advice of your pediatrician. During the visits to your pediatrician, your doctor will determine whether your baby can control the movements of his head and whether his reflex to suckle has changed to the swallowing movement. Your baby will begin to produce more saliva after month two, but the fact that he's drooling is proof he has yet to learn how to swallow.

Giving your baby cereals or solid foods before he's ready can not only damage his digestive system but may also lead to asthma or other illnesses and allergies down the road. Despite the dangers, many parents ignore this rule. According to one study, nearly three of every ten parents give their children solid food before the four- to six-month window. Also try to avoid starting your baby on fruit juices too quickly. The American Pediatric Academy recommends waiting until after six months.

Many Latina mothers believe in the myth that feeding babies cereal at night will make them sleep longer. It's an appealing idea after weeks and months of waking up in the middle of the night; however, it's not true. Cereals should be given to your baby in the form of baby food, not added to the bottle. Some Latina mothers like to add, on top of cereals, sugar or other foods to the bottle to give the milk more taste. This is not recommended because:

- Your baby can become obese from eating too many calories;
- You're not teaching your baby how to eat healthily (babies prefer naturally sweet tastes); and
- It can cause cavities.

By giving your infant cereal in the form of baby food, you're allowing him to control when he wants to stop eating. If the cereal is mixed with milk in the bottle, the extra calories are swallowed; your baby, who still needs to suckle, can't refuse it as he could do when he is being spoon-fed with solid food.

When your pediatrician says you can begin feeding your baby cereal, start with one type only, such as rice cereal (avoid wheat or corn cereal until age one since they may cause allergies). Then you can move on to other baby foods such as oats or barley that are fortified with iron. Avoid the baby foods that are mixed flavors, because they contain corn, and your baby's digestive system can't yet handle it. It's normal for your baby to reject baby food at first; it's new and very different from milk. Don't force your baby to eat solid foods, but at the same time don't give up and resort to adding them to the bottle. Just try again later. Feed your baby while he is sitting in a high chair, not when he is reclined, to avoid choking.

You can continue breastfeeding even when you begin to give your baby solid food. (The American Academy of Pediatrics recommends breastfeeding for the first year.) Your milk has all the nutrients your baby needs and the baby cereal is the perfect complement to mother's milk from four to six months. At this age babies breastfeed from four to six times a day.

Also, to avoid extra calories, you should use just your own milk or formula to mix the cereal, and not add sugar, honey, or other ingredients.

From Five to Seven Months: Vegetable and Fruit Purées

At five months to six months, if your baby has learned how to eat from a spoon and can control his head movements, your pediatrician may recommend that you feed your baby vegetable purées.

The easiest vegetable purées for your baby to digest are the ones colored yellow, such as sweet potato, pumpkin, or carrot (don't use corn; at this stage it may cause gas and allergies). Green vegetable purées like green beans or peas are also good. Try to alternate between the yellow and green vegetables. The yellow ones tend to be sweeter and you want your baby to learn to like different flavors of food. Another good idea: Give your baby only one type of vegetable for two or three days in a row. That way if your baby develops some type of allergy, you'll know what's causing the reaction. If all goes well with the vegetables, you can move on to fruit purées a few weeks later apples, bananas, peaches, or pears. Again, give your baby a few days with each fruit to see if any allergic reactions appear. You can buy the purées already mixed from the store or you can make your own. However, never add sugar or salt to either.

Regarding fruit juices, according to the American Academy of Pediatrics you can start giving them to your baby at six months, but it's a good idea to be cautious with them. At this stage we're trying to teach our babies how to eat healthily, and even though drinking fruit juice is good for your baby, you want to teach him to enjoy the fruit itself too. Also, it's very important to make the distinction between natural fruit juice and sugared juice. According to a recent study, juices and sugared drinks are the biggest contributors to calories in babies' diets. Also, Latino children have more cavities than any other group of children in the United States and too many sugared fruit drinks are partly to blame. It is important to remember not to give your baby fruit juices from the bottle; wait until he can drink from a cup.

AGE-APPROPRIATE FOODS AND PORTIONS

If you're breastfeeding your baby, you should continue feeding her from four to six times a day; if your baby gets formula, she should eat between twenty-four and thirty-six ounces a day.

When you first begin to give your baby solid foods, don't change your breastfeeding or formula schedule; just add in a couple of solid meals a day. But later, when your baby reaches six or seven months and can easily tolerate cereals, fruits, and vegetables, give your baby three meals a day with the breast milk or formula in between. Measure the purée with a spoon into a small dish and use a plastic baby spoon to feed your baby. The following table shows a sample menu for babies between five and seven months old that you can adapt to your own schedule. If you're breastfeeding, continue to breastfeed between four and six times a day, or more if your baby wants it.

This is an example of a menu for a child between the ages of five to seven months:

	Group	Serving	Food
Breakfast	Milk	6–8 ounces	Formula or breastfeeding
	Grain	1–3 spoonfuls	Oat cereal
	Fruit	1–3 spoonfuls	Apple compote
Midmorning snack	Milk	6–8 ounces	Formula or breastfeeding
	Grain	1–3 spoonfuls	Barley cereal
Lunch	Vegetable	1–3 spoonfuls	Sweet potato purée
	Fruit	1–3 spoonfuls	Peach compote
Afternoon snack	Milk	6–8 ounces	Formula or breastfeeding
	Grain	1–3 spoonfuls	Rice cereal
Dinner	Vegetable	1–3 spoonfuls	Carrot purée
	Fruit	1–3 spoonfuls	Banana compote
After dinner snack	Milk	6–8 ounces	Formula or breastfeeding

The vegetable and fruit purées you can choose from include:

Vegetables: Sweet potato, potato, pumpkin, carrot, peas, green beans

Fruits: Apple, peach, pear, banana, apricot

At this age, you can give your child small amounts of water (between four and eight ounces), depending on the climate where you live, but always use a cup. At first, your baby will do little more than spill the water. However, it's much better for your baby to learn now than to still be drinking from a bottle at twelve months.

Never force your baby to eat. A baby knows when he's had enough. Don't use food as a punishment or reward because that can lead to eating disorders. And remember, your baby doesn't have to be *gordito* to be healthy. Your pediatrician is the best source for you to find out if your baby's weight and size are on target.

From Seven to Nine Months: Soft Foods

Starting at seven to eight months, you can begin to replace the purées with other types of soft foods, such as:

- Mashed potatoes or lentil/bean purée.
- Vegetables and fruits cooked until they're soft.
- Soft, well-cooked meats (chicken, turkey, beef).
- Cottage cheese and yogurt.
- Bread or pieces of flour tortillas.

Your baby is still too young for certain foods: citrus fruits (oranges and lemons), eggs, chocolate, or tomatoes. Wait until nine months or more to give your baby these foods. Also don't give him foods that can cause choking such as pieces of hot dog, dried fruits, raisins, or grapes.

Patience is a virtue in this stage of your baby's development, because he will probably spend more time playing with his food than eating it. You will need a double serving of patience if you are a *madre muy pulcra*, a very tidy mother, since it's likely that you're now going to have to deal with pieces of spaghetti on the wall, in his hair, or any number of unusual places that are bound to strike your neatness nerve.

Fortunately this is just a stage. Neat mothers will just have to bite the bullet and prepare themselves for a messy few months of eating.

AGE-APPROPRIATE PORTIONS AND FOODS

Breastfed babies now eat between three and five times a day; formula-fed babies eat between twenty-four and thirty-two ounces a day. You can now give your baby between six and eight ounces of water a day from a cup. Even though fruit juices aren't really necessary at this age, you can give your baby between four and six ounces a day if you like. But make sure the fruit juice is natural, without added sugar. And remember to use a cup, not the bottle.

At this age, your baby will normally eat about five spoonfuls of vegetables and fruits at one sitting. But again, let your baby decide when he's full; never force-feed your baby. Offer your baby a variety of foods; let him play with the food with his fingers and decide what he likes and how much he wants to eat.

This is a sample menu for a baby seven to nine months:

	Group	Serving	Food
Breakfast	Milk	6–8 ounces	Formula or breastfeeding
	Grain	3–5 spoonfuls	Oat cereal
	Fruit	2–4 spoonfuls	Apple compote
Midmorning snack	Milk	6–8 ounces	Formula or breastfeeding
	Grain	3–5 spoonfuls	Barley cereal
Lunch	Grain/ Legume	3–6 spoonfuls	Lentil purée
	Protein	2–5 spoonfuls	Soft, cooked chicken
	Fruit	2–4 spoonfuls	Peach compote

	Group	Serving	Food
Afternoon snack	Milk	6–8 ounces	Formula or breastfeeding
	Grain or fruit	1–2 small units 2–4 spoonfuls	Baby crackers, soft bread, or pear compote
Dinner	Vegetable	3–5 spoonfuls	Carrots cooked until they're soft
	Protein	2–5 spoonfuls	Cottage cheese
After-dinner snack	Milk	6–8 ounces	Formula or breastfeeding

In addition to all this, remember your baby will continue to breast-feed three to five times a day. The foods you can choose from during these months include:

Cereals: Rice, oats, barley, or a mixture.

Grains and beans: Lentil or bean purée, peas, pasta, bread, toast, cookies, crackers, and low to moderate added sugar dry cereals (Cheerios, for instance).

Puréed or soft, cooked vegetables: Carrots, potatoes, sweet potatoes, pumpkin, green beans.

Puréed or soft, cooked fruits: Apple, orange, pear, peach, banana, fig, plum.

Proteins (meats and dairy): Chicken, fish (no shellfish), ground beef, boiled egg yolk, cottage cheese, yogurt.

From Nine to Twelve Months: More Consistent Meals

Between nine months and a year, your baby may begin to eat less because doing so expends less energy. Some babies eat only one full meal a day, and the rest of the day just pick a few things from their plate. Nevertheless, you should still try to establish an eating routine for your baby; don't let him eat a little of this and nibble on some of that all day long.

Many mothers worry during this stage; they think their babies *no comen nada*, aren't eating anything. Other babies get fixated on certain foods, and won't eat anything else. Relax. If your pediatrician says your baby is gaining the right amount of weight, if the food he's eating is healthy and nutritious, and he appears content and alert, there's no reason to worry. This is just another stage and the only thing you can do is make sure you offer him good, healthy foods several times a day. However, don't give in to the temptation to give your baby sugared drinks or sweets under the guise of "*al menos come algo,* at least he's eating something." It's better to stick to what is healthy for your baby. Even though it may not seem as though your baby is eating very much, if he is not sick, and as long as there are healthy foods around, you can rest assured your baby will not starve.

> No entiendo, *I can't understand how he can have so much energy, eating so little! Before he was eating much better. Now I worry if his growth will not be affected by this lack of appetite.*
> —Nuria, thirty-two years old

Latina mothers in particular have a difficult time with this stage when babies *no comen nada,* don't eat much. We all wonder what's gone wrong, whether our babies are going to be healthy for the rest of their lives because they aren't getting the proper nutrition now. Try to tell yourself this is only a stage, and just like many other things in your baby's life, this too will pass. Many unhealthy eating habits are formed during this stage, because mothers can't resist giving their baby just one little piece of candy or cookie: "After all, she has barely eaten anything all day." But if you do that, you're only beginning a vicious cycle. The more snacks you give her between meals to compensate for her lack of appetite at the last mealtime, the less she will eat at the next one. Around and around it goes. And so, inadvertently you may be overfeeding your baby not very healthy foods although you think "*apenas si come,* she is barely eating anything." Some advice on feeding your child during this stage:

- Sit the baby in his high chair so he can eat with the rest of the family. You can now begin to teach your baby how to use a baby spoon, or at least allow him to grab it while eating. At the table, the baby can begin to share some of the food the rest of the family is eating.

- Don't give your baby honey until she reaches one year because it can cause an illness called botulism. Don't give your baby peanuts or shellfish until she reaches one year, as they can cause severe allergies.

- Be careful with foods such as grapes, raisins, corn kernels, beans, candy, hot dogs, or any other type of food that may cause choking. Always stay close to your baby when he eats so you can help him if he begins to choke.

- Favor baby foods cooked at home over prepared baby dinners. They usually contain more calories, sodium, and preservatives. In this stage, your baby can usually enjoy the same foods the rest of the family eats.

- Always give your baby water to drink (four to eight ounces a day).

- Let your baby decide how much she wants to eat. Don't turn meals into battles or force your baby to eat. Even though you (or a grandmother or aunt) might think your baby isn't quite *gordito* enough, trust your pediatrician. Your pediatrician will let you know whether everything's okay with your baby's weight and growth. If you relax about the food, you will be teaching your baby not to obsess about what she eats—she will learn how to manage her own appetite and avoid eating too much in the future.

AGE-APPROPRIATE PORTIONS AND FOODS

At this age, your baby can begin to use his fingers to eat some of the following foods:

- Apples that are peeled and cut into pieces of eight.
- Soft cheeses.
- Well-cooked pasta or noodles.
- Little strips of fish, chicken, or turkey.

This is an example of a menu for a child between the ages of nine and twelve months:

	Group	Serving	Food
Breakfast	Milk	6–9 ounces	Formula or breastfeeding
	Grain	¼–½ cup	2–4 ounces cold cereal with low to moderate sugar (Cheerios, etc.)
	Fruit	½ cup	4 ounces apple cut into cubes

	Group	Serving	Food
Midmorning snack	Milk Fruit or grain	6–9 ounces ¼–½ cup	Formula or breastfeeding 2–4 ounces cold cereal with low to moderate sugar or cantaloupe cut into cubes
Lunch	Grain/Legume	¼–½ cup	2–4 ounces rice
	Protein: poultry, beef, fish, etc.	1–2 spoonfuls	Soft, cooked chicken
	Fruit	¼–½ piece	Banana
Afternoon snack	Milk Fruit or grain	6–9 ounces ¼–½ cup	Formula or breastfeeding 2–4 ounces cold cereal with low to moderate sugar or an apple or pear cut into cubes
Dinner	Vegetable	½ cup	4 ounces cooked pumpkin
	Protein: Poultry, fish, cheese, etc.	1–2 spoonfuls	Chopped turkey
	Fruit	¼–½ cup	Pears cut into cubes
After-dinner snack	Milk	6–9 ounces	Formula or breastfeeding

If you're breastfeeding your baby, you'll still need to do so three to four times a day.

The foods you can give your baby at this age are:

Cereals: It's no longer necessary to give your child baby food cereals; you can now give him dry low to moderate added sugar cereal such as puffed corn or Cheerios, etc.

Grains and legumes: Corn or flour tortillas (check for tolerance), whole wheat tortilla, whole wheat bread, noodles, rice, lentil or bean purées.

Fruits: Apple, pear, banana, cantaloupe, watermelon, orange, or pretty much any kind of fruit. But be careful your baby doesn't choke on grapes or raisins. Peel the grapes and remove the seeds. Also watch to see how well your baby tolerates acidic fruits such as strawberries and kiwis since they can cause allergies.

Vegetables: Carrot, pumpkin, peas, broccoli, green beans, etc. You can give your baby pretty much any type of vegetable that's been cooked until it's soft.

Proteins (meats and dairy): Ground beef, pork, chicken, fish (not shellfish), egg whites, soft cheeses (white cheese, etc.) tofu.

The Menu Between One and Two Years Old: Eating Any Kind of Food

If you're still breastfeeding, you're probably breastfeeding your baby three times a day or less. At this age you can stop breastfeeding or giving him formula and switch to whole cow's milk. Don't give your baby skim milk because whole cow's milk has nutrients your baby needs to grow until he reaches the age of two. Children one to two years old will drink sixteen to twenty-four ounces of milk per day. Try to give him the milk in a cup. It's important to wean your baby now from the bottle. Also, at eighteen months, you can cut back on the iron-fortified cereals. Your baby can now eat cold or warm cereals without difficulty. Still, try to avoid cereals that have too much added sugar.

Ideally, a one- to two-year-old child will eat three times a day (breakfast, lunch, and dinner) with two snacks in between meals. Nevertheless, not all children will eat that much and it's normal for them to have an irregular appetite. Instead of worrying about how much your child eats each day, focus on how much is eaten over the entire week and how nutritious that food is. It's also normal for many children to eat one type of food over and over again. Don't give up. Keep offering your child a variety of healthy foods. This phase will also pass. A visit to the pediatrician is the best way to assure yourself that your child is eating and growing normally.

It's a good idea to have a meal with the entire family together at least once a day. Children learn from adults and if all of you are eating the same foods, it's more probable that your baby will try them. That's also the way children learn table manners. Let your child give it a shot with infant plastic forks and spoons.

Is Your Child Lactose Intolerant?

If your doctor tells you your child is lactose intolerant (intolerant to milk products' natural sugar), your child can still enjoy the nutritional benefits of these foods:

- Offer him yogurt: Yogurt with active cultures contains less lactose.

- Serve cheese in his sandwiches, salads, or other foods: Cheeses are naturally low in lactose.

- Serve small portions of milk with his favorite foods; such as during lunch or dinnertime. Other foods can improve your child's ability to break down lactose.

- Consider offering your child lactose-reduced or lactose-free milk and other dairy foods. And remember to always talk to your pediatrician or nutritionist if you suspect your child has a food intolerance or an allergy.

AGE-APPROPRIATE PORTIONS AND FOODS

At one or two years, you can now give your child foods such as whole eggs, raw vegetables, and new types of legumes. Present these different foods to your child at the beginning of the meal, when he's hungrier. Start off with a small piece, but don't force him to eat.

This is an example of a menu for a child between the ages of one and two:

	Group	Serving	Food
Breakfast	Dairy	½ cup	4 ounces whole cow's milk
	Grain	¼–½ cup	2–4 ounces cold cereal, low to moderate sugar (Cheerios, etc.)
	Fruit	½ cup	4 ounces melon cut into cubes
Midmorning snack	Dairy	½–¾ cup	4–6 ounces yogurt (not fat-free)
	Grains	½ slice of bread, or 3 crackers	Whole wheat bread or 3 crackers

	Group	Serving	Food
Lunch	Vegetable	½ cup	4 ounces raw carrots with chopped tomato
	Meat: Beef, poultry, fish, etc.	1–2 spoonfuls	Chicken cooked until it's soft
	Fruit	¼–½ cup	Banana
Afternoon snack	Dairy	½–¾ cup or 1 ounce	4–6 ounces yogurt (not fat-free), or 1 ounce natural cheese
	Fruit or grain	¼–½ cup	Apple or pear cut into cubes or sugarless cold cereal
Dinner	Vegetable	¼–½ cup	2–4 ounces broccoli
	Meat: Beef, poultry, fish, eggs, etc.	1 egg	1 egg (omelet)
	Grain/ legume	⅓–½ cup	3–4 ounces rice or pasta

Your child can now eat pretty much any kind of food, but be careful with popcorn, grapes, pieces of hot dogs, and other things that could lead to choking. Never leave your child alone to eat. Some recommended foods from each food group are:

Milk and milk products: Whole cow's milk, regular yogurt with fat (not diet), cottage cheese with fat (not fat-free), soft cheeses

Vegetables: Broccoli, green beans, spinach, lettuce, carrots, corn, pumpkin, peppers, or pretty much any other vegetable, as tolerated

Fruits: Apple, orange, pear, banana, peach, canned fruits that don't have much sugar, or pretty much any other fruit

Grains: Lentils, beans, garbanzos, peas, rice, pasta, tortillas, bread, or any other grain or legume

Proteins: Beef, chicken, fish, whole egg

Adiós, Baby Bottle!

It's very common for Latino families to feed their babies with a bottle well past twelve months. Some even push it until the child is four or five! Mothers fear their babies will stop drinking milk and will be deprived of the nutrients found in milk if they do away with the bottle.

> *The only way I am able to make Cristina have her milk is in the bottle. I know she is maybe too big for the bottle, but I don't want her to stop drinking her milk.*
>
> —Susana, twenty-nine years old

But there are several reasons why pediatricians say at twelve months it's time to say *hasta là vista,* good-bye, bottle.

- *Obesity:* One of those reasons has to do with obesity. According to a scientific study, children older than eighteen months who still feed from a bottle or who drink other types of sweet liquids several times a day are more likely to become obese. A bottle of milk contains about 180 calories, maybe more for Latino babies because their mothers usually add cereals, sugar, honey, or other high-calorie ingredients. If you add those "bottle calories" to the calories already in the solid meals, your baby is eating more than she needs. Another negative effect of bottle feeding: Your baby may lose her appetite at mealtime. This in turn makes parents worry and wonder why the baby won't eat.

- *Anemia*: Bottle feeding also means your baby will get too much calcium. Excessive calcium interferes with the absorption of iron, which can result in anemia. One study showed that children who continue to feed from a bottle are more likely to be anemic.

- *Cavities*: One thing parents really need to avoid is giving their baby a bottle while he lies in bed at night. The sugars in the milk will stay on the baby's teeth through the night, which may cause cavities. Also, you need to start "brushing" your baby's teeth at an early age. Latino children have more cavities than any other group of children in the United States. Adding sugar or honey to milk to get your baby to drink more of it is a bad idea. Honey can cause allergies, and sugar, just like honey or high-sugared cereals, doesn't do anything more than add extra calories to your baby's diet. Plus it ruins teeth. Remember, milk has its own type of sugar, called lactose; you don't need to add anything to make it taste good.

As children grow, it becomes more and more difficult to wean them off the bottle, especially if they've gotten used to it to fall sleep. The sooner you teach your child to drink from a cup, the easier it will be to say good-bye to the baby bottle.

And if you've been breastfeeding your baby all the way up to twelve months, switch directly to whole cow's milk in a cup. You don't need to give him formula after twelve months of age.

The Obese Infant

After reading all this, you may still be wondering if your child is obese. The best person to ask is your pediatrician. Pediatricians have charts and tables that define what a child should weigh according to its size and age. These charts are divided into sections called percentiles. If your child is in the 85th to 95th percentile or higher, that's a case of obesity. In the Appendix you will find sample growth charts similar to what your pediatrician will use.

Your baby has a greater chance of becoming obese in the future if you had gestational diabetes, if you gained a lot of weight during the last trimester of pregnancy, or if your family has a history of obesity. If one of these situations applies to you, you need to be more aware of how your baby is growing because he might have weight problems later on.

The period from birth to two years is when parents should take special care to avoid obesity for several reasons:

- This time period is when many Latinos believe a "*bebé gordo es un bebé sano,* a fat baby is a healthy baby," and it's easier to overlook the warning signs of obesity.

- Children who are obese at this age are more likely to be obese as adults.

- This is the time when children learn to eat and begin to form the eating habits (good and bad) they'll use for the rest of their lives.

If your pediatrician determines that your baby is obese, don't go running for a "miracle diet." Putting a child on a diet in this stage of its development can stunt its growth. The American Medical Association recommends that children younger than two get half of their daily calories from fat to ensure proper brain development. Instead of focusing so much on how much your baby eats, try to focus on how well your baby eats: *Calidad, no cantidad,* quality, not quantity. The standards given in this chapter of how much your child should eat at the different stages of its development are good general models to follow. Your baby will have a structured diet based on healthy foods that will help your child grow without excessive calories.

Latino Feeding Traditions to Watch for in an Obese Infant

If your child is obese, aside from watching the kind of foods he gets, you need to be aware of certain attitudes toward food that your child may hold. For example, it's common among Latino families for grandparents to give their grandchildren treats such as candy or great-tasting fatty foods such as hot dogs or french fries, which are appropriate to give only occasionally to the obese child, or any child.

> *Pedro is my only* nieto, granchild. *How can I say no when he looks at me with that chubby smile, and says, "*Abuelita, quiero un dulce, Grandma, I want some sweets"? *My son tells me that I am spoiling him, but isn't that what* abuelitas *are for?*
>
> —Nora, sixty-three years old

Sometimes it's difficult for people from past generations to understand that obese children need limits on their diets. Talk to those grandparents. Explain how you're working with your pediatrician or nutritionist to create a healthy future for your child. Take your mother or your aunt with you on the next visit to the pediatrician so the doctor can explain the problems and consequences of being overweight for a child.

Another attitude to watch out for is using food as a calming device. Be careful about giving candy to your child when he's crying or using food as a reward or punishment. If you give food to your child when he's crying or you use food as a reward, your child may begin to confuse feelings of frustration or anger with the need to eat.

Physical Activity

Movement and exercise are a normal part of daily life for children this age, because they're learning how their bodies work as they move from crawling to walking. So encourage your child to move around. Baby strollers, baby seats, and other contraptions we use to keep our babies from moving around do help us keep an eye on them (and give us some welcome moments of peace), but they also restrict their movements. The best thing to do for your child is to create a safe zone where movement and exploration is allowed. The more time children can spend in a safe space where they can move around, the better they'll use their muscles and promote their development.

Encouraging children to exercise at an early age helps them learn good, healthy habits that they'll follow for the rest of their lives. Children young and old look to their parents for examples of how to exercise. For example, if children see the family regularly going for afternoon walks at the park, they will consider that as normal. But if families spend every afternoon sitting on the couch watching TV, the children will learn that's normal, and getting outside for exercise will become out of the ordinary.

Changing our exercise routine can be tough, especially if we arrive home tired after a long day's work. But think of it this way: A small child is the perfect excuse to make changes in our lifestyle. Children watch what we parents do, they emulate us. Going for a walk with children gives them and you time in the fresh air (sun helps our skin make vitamin D), burns calories, and offers a chance to socialize with other children and their parents.

All those fancy baby gyms aren't really necessary for a child's growth and development; that is, you don't need to spend money on your child's exercise. However, those gyms do provide parents an opportunity to meet other parents who are interested in promoting their children's physical activity.

And play a lot with your children: tickle them, let them crawl on the floor, put a toy across the room and have them work to get it. Associating exercise with fun is a great way to teach children to enjoy physical activity.

7

Nutrition from Ages Two to Five

Not all parents who come to my office are worried about their two- to five-year-old children being overweight. In fact, some parents come because they think their child "has stopped eating" and they don't understand why.

I never had problems with her eating. She had a great appetite when she was an infant and gobbled up everything I gave her! Now she won't try any new food. Some days, it seems she won't eat anything. What's happening to my baby?

—Jackeline, twenty-four years old

What's happening to this "baby" and to many others is that they're not babies anymore. The rapid growth your child went through during the first two years of life has slowed down. Between ages two and five, children develop socially, intellectually, and emotionally, but the physical growth slows down. That lessens a child's interest in food and also may decrease the appetite. During the preschool phase, it's especially important for parents to establish healthy eating habits for their children so as to prevent obesity. There are several reasons for this:

Children lose their ability to control their appetites if parents or caretakers pressure them to eat when they're not hungry.
Different studies have shown that children between the ages of three and five instinctively know to eat daily only what they need to grow without getting fat. For example, if children eat a big lunch, they'll automatically eat a lighter dinner. However, this natural regulation mechanism disappears if parents force children to eat a predetermined portion. Parents shouldn't try to override what their children's bodies are telling them is enough food. If your children say they've had enough, listen to them; don't force them to eat because you'll interfere with their natural appetite-regulating mechanism. Nor should parents abandon a healthy menu in favor of sweets and candies just so the kids will "eat something." If your children lose their capacity to regulate their own appetites, in future years they'll eat without knowing how to stop. Of course, the inability to stop eating can lead to obesity. A study done on preschool children showed that overweight children had less capacity to determine when they were not hungry and therefore didn't know when to stop eating. Using food as a reward or as punishment can also interfere with children's ability to regulate their own appetites and recognize when they're full.

It's best to divide up the responsibilities. Let's say the parents are responsible for presenting the children with a variety of healthy foods (like the ones you'll find in the sample menus in the following pages) and the child is responsible for deciding how much of those foods to eat. This system may be a little difficult for the Latino parent who's convinced that a *gordito* or chubby child is a healthy child. And it can be especially difficult for parents (like the example of the mother at the beginning of the chapter) who worry that their children aren't eating enough and feel the need to pressure the children to eat more. As a pediatric dietician, I can assure you there's nothing to worry about: Even if your children aren't eating as much as you think they should, as long as you offer them a variety of healthy foods to eat, they're not going to starve or suffer nutritional deficiencies that affect their development. Just consider how much the science of nutrition has advanced in recent years. For example, in most industrialized countries, it was once thought that formula was better for babies than breast milk. Today we know that's absolutely false. By the same token, we also now know that it's not a good idea to force children to clean their plates because it interferes with their natural regulation mechanisms. Making children eat more than they want causes more problems than it solves.

Children between the ages of two and five begin to learn what foods they like; family influences those tastes.
We're all born with an appetite for sweets and salty foods. Aside from that, all the foods we like are acquired tastes. Children learn to like the foods familiar to them—the foods their parents, siblings, relatives, and classmates eat. So setting an example is important. If you or your partner or other members of the family often eat fried foods, fatty meats, and sweets, your child will probably not develop an appetite for vegetables or whole grains. Healthy eating is a family issue.

Children will also learn to like foods that are presented to them as rewards. Sweets and fatty foods, which so many children like, are often used as a reward for good behavior or for having eaten a different food that's considered healthier. Who hasn't told a child: "You can have your *postre*, dessert, if you finish your vegetables"? But this tactic only encourages the child to prefer dessert to vegetables; plus it teaches the child that food is a game or a competition, and not about nutrition. I recommend that parents instruct children on the order of how food should be eaten. For example: "You will first eat your vegetables and then your dessert," instead of making dessert a reward for eating something else first. We Latinos are used to having our meals end with flan or a piece of cake. Dessert isn't really necessary, unless it's a way to provide fruit or yogurt, something sweet and healthy.

You will have great influence over what foods your child likes by:

- the foods you make available to your child,
- the time you eat your meals,
- the foods children see you, their siblings, or sitters eating,
- the way you use food (as a reward, punishment, or as a celebration).

A phase called adiposity rebound occurs as children get closer to five years of age. Children who enter the adiposity rebound phase earlier are more likely to become obese adults.

Right around five years of age, children's weight drops, and then begins to increase again. This dip in body mass is known as adiposity rebound. The sooner a child enters this phase, the greater the chance of obesity later in that child's life. In girls, when the adiposity rebound phase hits early, it results in a greater weight later on. No one really knows why some children enter this period sooner than others, but it's believed to be a combination of genetics and environment. So even though you can't change a child's genes, it is possible to alter eating habits that could lead to obesity.

Having an obese parent is one of the factors that can predict an early entry into the adiposity rebound phase. If this applies to your family, you should contact your pediatrician or nutritionist so he or she can monitor your child in case this adiposity rebound stage comes early. Consulting a pediatrician or nutritionist is really important for Latino parents, because several studies have shown we Latinos have a different definition of what it means for children to be obese. Latino parents often think their two- to six-year-old children aren't overweight, when in fact they are.

From Two to Three Years: The *No!* Phase

Right around two years of age, children begin to realize they're little independent people in their own right. And what better way to show that independence than by doing exactly the opposite of what a parent says!

> *It seems that* no! *is the only word in her vocabulary lately. Meals used to be a pleasant time for us, but that's history now!*
>
> *—Antonio, thirty-one years old*

Parents must remember no matter how disagreeable a two-year-old is, that isn't necessarily how that child will act as a teenager and adult. The "terrible twos" period—full of *no!*—is just a normal stage of development and a necessary one for children to become their own people.

Two-year-olds are famous for refusing to try new foods (sometimes they'll even reject the foods they know), especially the healthy ones, such as fruits and vegetables. Moreover, this is the age when children will grow out of using diapers. This can cause them anxiety, and may affect their appetite. In many families, this is also the time when the little brother or sister comes along. The arrival of a new member of the family can also affect your two-year-old's attitude toward eating; sometimes children will express their conflicting emotions by not eating.

All those factors, plus the fact that two-year-olds naturally eat less because their bodies don't grow as quickly, are enough to see why eating can be quite an emotional drama.

DINNER TABLE WARS

Even though it's normal for children to seem uninterested in food or for them to refuse to eat certain things, that doesn't mean it's easy for parents to deal with. Many parents run out of patience every evening at the dinner table, fighting *las batallas en la mesa*, the dinner table wars. Just keep in mind this phase will pass and remember which of the two of you is the adult. More than anything try to avoid the dinner table wars; no one really wins and they can reinforce bad eating habits.

It's important not to threaten. One survey of Latino parents of pre-school children showed the most common threats were:

- We'll give you a shot.
- You'll need a laxative.
- Your father will spank you when he gets home.
- We're going to leave you home alone.
- I'll love your brother/sister more than you.

Even though they may not eat everything, as long as you offer your children a variety of healthy foods, they won't die of hunger or become malnourished. The best you can do for your children is let them eat the amount they want, and respect what their bodies are telling them they need to eat.

REJECTING NEW FOODS

One of Dr. Seuss's most famous stories is *Green Eggs and Ham*. In this story, a cat tries over and over again, page after page, to get the protagonist to try some green eggs and ham. The protagonist refuses every time. Finally, after much begging, the protagonist agrees to try, just a little bit. And at that moment, his whole attitude changes. He loves green eggs and ham, and it becomes one of his favorite dishes.

During the "terrible twos," children often apply their favorite word—*no!*—to new foods, especially vegetables. Your strategy as a parent should be to mimic the cat in the story: have patience, persevere, and try to keep a sense of humor. In fact, children saying no to a new food isn't the stuff of Dr. Seuss stories, it's real. One survey found that parents need to offer their children a certain food between eight and ten times before they'll consider accepting it.

When you give your child something new, start out by saying, "Just take a little bite to see if you like it." Don't insist your child finish the whole thing. And don't forget to praise your children when they do try something new. The best way to introduce something new is to present it with something familiar. And remember, if you don't eat vegetables and other healthy foods that you want your children to eat, it will be unlikely that they will want to eat them.

For children this age, familiarizing themselves with new foods means touching and playing with their food. Have a little patience with this food play, because it's normal, and beyond that, it helps children accept the novelty of the different tastes and textures.

SCHEDULES AND LIMITS

Children this age are constantly pushing to see how much they can get away with. They're searching to find limits or boundaries. Establishing limits and creating a structure or schedule for the day are key to fostering good behavior in children. That also applies to how children deal with food. Routines—doing things the same way every day—help children feel more secure. For example, dinnertime and bedtime are closely related. If your children have a set bedtime (and they sleep enough), they'll wake up at about the same time every day, and have breakfast at the same time every day. With that done, the rest of the meals of the day will also fall into place at about the same times every day. That way, parents can plan a menu with three full meals a day, along with one to three snacks. On the other hand, if your children go to bed at a different time every night, they'll also wake up at different times (or they'll be very tired). And that will affect how much they want to eat and when.

When you establish these rules, make sure you remember what you've said, because children will always push to make sure you're still enforcing them. For example, if your rule is to eat at the kitchen table, not watching television, stay firm and say no every time your child asks to watch cartoons during dinner. When you give in, you only create confusion.

One way to avoid saying no so much is to give your child options to choose from. For example, if your children insist on eating standing up, you might say: "You know we're all supposed to eat sitting down.

Do you want to eat in the kitchen or in the dining room?" Or if your children want to watch television while they eat, you could say: "You know we're not to watch television while we eat, but I'll sit with you here and eat. Would you like to tell me about how your day at school was, or would you rather I tell you a story?" And every time your child does something you've asked, don't forget to praise. That's one of the best ways to encourage right behavior.

Even though your children may still be young, it's really not too early to begin establishing limits and healthy habits. In older children, these are some of the behaviors that can help fight obesity:

- Limit the time your children watch television or play computer games. More than two hours a day is too much.

- Don't let your children get used to drinking soft drinks. Soda contributes greatly to obesity in children and teenagers. Water is always the best drink. According to a study, children at this age who drink more than nine ounces of soda a day are more likely to drink less than eight ounces of milk daily. Less milk equals less calcium, an essential mineral for young children.

- Get your children used to brushing their teeth after every meal and before going to bed. Latino children have more cavities than any others in the United States.

DAY CARE: TAKE FOOD FROM HOME OR EAT THERE?

More than half of working women today have young children. And according to census data, a majority of those children spend time in day care. Some day care centers require parents to send their children in with food from home. Others allow parents to pay a little extra to have their children eat food prepared at the center. Some centers allow you to choose between the two options.

You'll have more control over what your children eat if you send them to day care with food prepared from home. It'll be cheaper too, although you will have to spend more time preparing the meals. You can plan a menu for the entire week or two ahead of time using the menu samples in this chapter. There are plenty of healthy and tasty dishes you can make ahead of time, and then freeze in smaller portions. Then all you'd have to add every day would be fruits, vegetables, and dairy. Stay on top of how your children are eating by asking the day care providers whether they're finishing their food, whether they're sharing it with others, or whether they're leaving a lot behind. You should also be aware of any rules the center has set up that limits what children can bring in from home. For example, if there's no limit on how many sodas or sweets children can bring, it's likely that leftovers from lunch will be shared among the rest of the children.

If your day care offers lunch sometimes it's difficult to decide if it's better to pack lunch than buying the one at the center. The first step in making that decision is finding out what food is on the menu at the center. The center must give you a list of what foods are served to the children and when. Compare the center's menu with the ones you find in this book to make sure there are enough fruits, vegetables, grains, and milk products in the day care meals. Also watch out for a menu high in sugar and fat.

Finally, remember it's our responsibility as parents to teach our children how to eat properly, even if they're buying lunch at the day care center. If you are not really happy with the food served at the center and you have no other choice, try to balance out your child's menus with what you prepare for her at home.

Talk often with your children about why it's important to eat vegetables, fruits, grains, and why they should avoid sugared drinks and sweets. If you do that in a language they can understand, you'll be teaching lessons they'll benefit from for the rest of their lives.

Menu for Children Ages Two to Three

A child at this age usually needs around 1,000 to 1,200 calories a day, that is, about half of what you probably eat per day. At this stage your child needs specific nutrients like calcium, proteins, vitamin A, and iron to develop properly. It is easier to concentrate on a diverse diet than to focus on your child's eating a specific food. For example, if your child doesn't like yams, you can give him a slice of cantaloupe because both foods contain vitamin A. If he doesn't like milk, you can give him other foods rich in calcium like cheese or yogurt.

Whole or regular milk should only be given to children until they are twenty-four months old. After they reach the age of two, any low-fat milk is fine ("low fat," 2 percent, 1 percent, or even skim), as long as your child is getting enough calories from other foods. Even if your child asks you to sweeten her milk, try not to do it because milk already has its own sugar, called lactose. Sugar will only add extra empty calories, with no nutrients. If you are sweetening the milk for your child, start decreasing the sugar little by little until she drinks milk in its natural form. But don't be extreme; your child can have sweetened milk, as well as flavored milks (chocolate and strawberry milk) from time to time. She will benefit just the same from the calcium and other nutrients found in milk. The idea is to keep your child from becoming dependent on sweeteners to drink something as common and healthy as "plain" milk.

Following is a sample daily menu for a child from age two to three years of age. The serving sizes are adjusted according to the Latino food pyramid in Chapter Four. The amounts of foods are distributed through the day. That is, one cup of vegetables can be divided into a half cup of vegetables at lunch and another half cup at dinner. The same goes for the other food groups, too.

DAILY SERVINGS FOR
CHILDREN TWO TO THREE YEARS OLD
Calories: 1,000 to 1,200 divided the following way:

Food group	Amount
Grains, legumes	2–2½ cups
Vegetables	¾ of a cup or more
Fruit	1–1½ cups/units
Low-fat dairy products	1½–2 cups
Lean meat	3–4 ounces
Healthy fats	1 tablespoon

Some examples of foods for each food group are:

Dairy products: 2 percent, 1 percent, or skim milk; yogurt, natural cheese, processed cheese, iced milk, pudding.

Vegetables: Carrots, squash, broccoli, spinach, romaine lettuce, green, yellow, and red vegetables. Any cooked or raw vegetable he tolerates in small bites.

Fruit: Apples, pears, bananas, melon, watermelon, oranges, kiwis, mangoes, papayas, breadfruit. Any fruits she tolerates, either fresh or cooked, in small bites.

Grains: Corn tortillas, white or whole rice, potatoes, yucca, yam, taro, breads, cereals, pastas, noodles, lentils, beans, quinoa.

Proteins: Lean meats including beef, pork, chicken, or fish (no shellfish), and eggs.*

---

*If you suspect an allergy to certain foods (eggs, peanuts, honey, strawberries, fish), you should talk to your pediatrician right away.

SAMPLE MENU FOR A CHILD TWO TO THREE YEARS OLD
(BETWEEN 1,000 TO 1,200 CALORIES)

	Group	Serving	Food
Breakfast	Dairy	½ cup	4 ounces 1% milk
	Grains	½ cup	4 ounces instant cereal
	Fruit	½ piece	½ banana
Midmorning snack (if available)	Grains	½ piece	½ corn or whole wheat tortilla
	Fat	1–2 teaspoons	Avocado or low-fat sour cream
	Fruit	½ cup	4 ounces natural juice
Lunch	Meat	2 ounces	Shredded chicken
	Grains	1 unit	1 slice whole wheat bread
	Vegetable	½ cup	4 ounces cooked broccoli
	Fat	½ teaspoon	Low-fat ranch dressing for the vegetables
	Dairy	½ cup	4 ounces 1% milk
Snack	Fruit	½ cup	4 ounces low-sugar canned peaches or fresh fruit
	Grain	½ unit	6 animal crackers

	Group	Serving	Food
Dinner	Grains	½ cup–1 cup	4–8 ounces spaghetti
	Meat	1 ounce (2 tablespoons)	Lean ground beef
	Vegetable	2 ounces (4 tablespoons)	Shredded carrots
	Dairy	½ cup	4 ounces low-fat yogurt
	Fruit	½ cup	4 ounces chopped strawberries in yogurt

At first glance the amount of foods might appear to be excessive; however, this sample menu includes the appropriate servings for all food groups, distributed throughout the day. Let your child decide how much he needs to eat. Refer to the Appendix for the daily calorie recommendations according to level of physical activity.

From Four Years to Five: I Want to Be a Grown-up

Children who have just turned four still have a little of the "terrible twos" in them, but they're beginning to calm down and take on adult behaviors. What a relief for parents! Also, children this age learn a new favorite word: "why?" They want to know why things happen and how to cooperate with others. Four-year-olds love watching adults do things, and then try to copy them. This is a great time to explain in more detail how foods are different and why they should eat vegetables and fruits.

Four-year-olds need a little help eating, but as they get closer to five, they can pretty much do it on their own. You'll find children this age love to have lengthy conversations at the dinner table—just as the adults do—so they make take forever to finish the food on their plates.

Even though at this age their appetites are pretty much stabilized, some days they may not be very hungry. So parents should continue to look at the big picture and monitor what their children eat in the course of a week, not daily.

IRON, ZINC, AND CALCIUM LEVELS

Vitamins and minerals are essential components for good health and development (see Chapter 3). But for children this age, there are three that require your special attention because they greatly influence the growth of your children, as well as how they perform in school.

Iron-deficiency anemia is common among preschool children and among Latino children in general. They don't have enough iron in their diets. Also, studies have made a connection between obesity and anemia due to insufficient iron.

In addition, without iron, our bodies can't make red blood cells, which means oxygen doesn't get to all parts of the body, including the brain. That's why it's always a good idea to include foods that are rich in iron, such as iron-fortified breads and cereals, beans, lentils, raisins, and dried peaches. Iron is absorbed much better if it's accompanied by vitamin C, which is found in natural orange juice, strawberries, broccoli, tomatoes, and mangos. Children who have an iron deficiency in their diets are—though not always—the ones who rarely eat meat, don't like iron-fortified cereals, and don't eat vegetables with iron. You can offer your child liver, beef, beans, nuts (with supervision to prevent choking), baked potatoes, oatmeal, and iron-fortified cereals. Your pediatrician might prescribe iron supplements if a blood test shows that your child has anemia.

The same thing happens with zinc. Some preschool children don't get enough zinc in their diets. This mineral plays a critical role in insulin production and may help in preventing diabetes, a disease that disproportionately affects Latinos. You'll find zinc in fish, legumes, whole cereals, red meat, nuts, tofu, and eggs.

According to one study, Latina preschool girls have the least amount of calcium in their diets. Calcium is crucial to building strong bones and teeth and other tissues. This mineral can be found in milk and milk products such as yogurt and cheese, as well as in green leafy vegetables such as spinach or broccoli. Fish such as canned sardines and salmon canned with bones also provide calcium. It's especially important to make sure children, especially girls, have enough calcium.

SNACKS

The appetite of four- and five-year-old children can change day by day. But if you stay on your schedule, you'll at least keep your children from eating at all hours. It's easy to give them more snacks just because they didn't eat all of breakfast or lunch. It's tempting, but all you're doing is making it harder for them to build up an appetite for the next meal. If children aren't hungry after eating a heavy snack, then they won't want to eat the fruits and vegetables you know they need to be healthy.

Make every effort to give your children natural and nutritious snacks. Avoid sweets or fried foods that contain a lot of fat, like doughnuts or potato chips. It's much better to serve up a small sandwich, a little bag of ready-to-eat carrots, or peeled fruit cut up into pieces. Natural fruit is always better than prepared juices, because children will feel fuller eating something solid.

Fifty years ago, orange juice was the number one fruit juice. Now children five and younger prefer apple juice. Even though it's low in fat and nutritious, the high amount of sugar in packaged apple juice can mean a huge number of calories. That's not all. Besides being high in sugar, juices can become a substitute for milk, which is never a good idea. So always choose natural fruit juices over prepackaged ones. If you have to use packaged ones, make sure they are 100 percent juice only. And make sure your children understand that eating fruits and other natural snacks is good for their health. Later on, the vending machines found in many middle and high schools can be a huge temptation. If your children develop a taste for healthy snacks, they'll make healthier choices in the future.

FAMILY MEALS

This is the time to begin eating as a family, if you haven't already. Between the ages of four and five, children can now sit in a chair with a booster or on a little pillow; they don't need a high chair.

Even though it may be more convenient to feed your children separately, at different times than the rest of the family, don't give in. Eating together is a great opportunity for children to learn table manners and get used to eating family foods. Another benefit: it's easier to introduce new foods to the family menu when everyone eats together, because younger children see what adults and older siblings eat. If your children don't really get too excited about trying new foods, don't worry. Just say they're missing out on something really tasty, and then offer it again on another occasion. Remember, you may need to give children eight to ten tries before they really take to something new.

Another benefit to the family meal is that it removes the television as the center of attention. Television is a distraction and diverts attention we should give to food. When an entire family eats together, they can review what's happened during the day and enjoy the company of other family members. If children begin to relate food with spending enjoyable time with family, they'll develop a positive and healthy attitude toward nutrition.

> When I was a girl my father was very strict about family dinners. Everybody had to be on time, clean hands, clean face. There was no TV then, just plática familiar, family conversation. Those dinners are actually one of the best memories I have from my childhood and I want my children to enjoy them too.
>
> —Margarita, thirty-eight years old

One last appeal for the family meal: Children who eat at least one meal a day with family follow a healthier diet than those who don't. Children who eat with family eat more fruits and vegetables and have higher levels of calcium, iron, folic acid, and vitamins B_6, B_{12}, C, and E.

RESTAURANT BEHAVIOR

Once children reach this age, it's much easier for them to behave like little adults when the family goes out to eat. But don't forget, they're still young.

To make sure eating out is a fun family experience, you can take the following precautions:

- Don't arrive at the restaurant with your children starving. A small healthy snack ahead of time will help them wait calmly until the food is served.

- Take some crayons and a notebook to allow your child to draw until the food arrives, or ask the restaurant for some if available.

- Explain to your children that they're now a little older, so they must act that way, and follow the rules of eating out by remembering all their table manners.

Menu for Children Ages Four to Five

At this age, your child's need for fats continues to drop (although it is important to eat the right amount of good fats for the rest of our lives). Children under two years old need half of the calories in their diets to come from fats, but after the age of two, this amount drops to 30 percent. Your child may drink milk with less fat in it now, like skim milk or one that has only 1 percent or 2 percent of fat. However, it is important to reduce the fat in other foods too. Some good ways to do this are:

- Adding fish to the diet, along with chicken, lean pork, and beef.
- Skinning chicken and trimming fat from all meats.
- Using healthier fats like olive oil and margarines free of trans fats instead of lard or shortening.
- Using "low-fat" methods of cooking like baking, broiling, poaching, or steaming.
- Serving foods high in fiber, including whole wheat breads, cereals, beans, legumes, and vegetables.

From age three on it is important to eat enough fiber because this can lower the risk of heart disease and cancer for your child in adulthood. But increasing fiber has to be done slowly. If your child isn't used to eating fiber-rich foods, these can cause gas or sudden abdominal bloating.

Something you don't want to forget is that your child needs to drink proper amounts of water, not only because it is essential for the body to work properly but because it lessens the initial symptoms of a fiber-rich diet.

Calcium is another nutritional priority at this age, because it means having strong bones later. Children at this age require a great deal of calcium every day. Some good sources of calcium are low-fat dairy products (like milk or cheese), tofu, salmon (cooked with bones), calcium-fortified drinks and juices, canned sardines, spinach, and ice cream (only occasionally served).

Candies and sweets may be one of your child's favorite things at this age. To prohibit them totally isn't an option because one way or the other, he will be exposed to them (and furthermore, this type of prohibition tends to produce just the opposite effect), but it is important to set limits. Children who eat sweets every day, or very frequently, tend to be inadequately nourished. You can set sweets aside for birthdays, parties, or special outings.

Caffeine should not be part of his diet at this age either because it is a stimulant that can interfere with his ability to concentrate or sleep. Avoid sodas and other drinks that contain caffeine, and, of course, coffee. In this day and age, there are many beverages made specifically for children that contain large quantities of caffeine. This is another reason why it is important to read the nutritional information labels on products to know what ingredients are in them.

If you offer your child a varied diet, she probably won't need a vitamin supplement, but it is important to check with your pediatrician to see if your child is anemic, something very common at this age. If she is anemic, her doctor or nutritionist will recommend a supplement for her.

DAILY SERVINGS FOR
CHILDREN AGES FOUR AND FIVE
Calories: 1,300 to 1,400 calories divided in the following way:

Food group	Amount
Grains, legumes	2½–3 cups/units
Vegetables	1½ cups or more
Fruit	2 cups/units
Low-fat dairy	2½–3 cups
Lean meats	4–6 ounces
Healthy fats	1–1½ tablespoons

Some examples of recommended foods from each group are:

Dairy products: 2 percent, 1 percent, or skim milk; yogurt, natural cheese, processed cheese, ice cream, pudding.

Vegetables: Tomatoes, carrots, squash, broccoli, spinach, romaine lettuce, cucumbers, onions, green onions, green, yellow, and red vegetables. Any raw or cooked vegetable that the family eats, cut in small bites.

Fruit: Apples, pears, bananas, melon, watermelon, oranges, kiwis, mangoes, papayas, breadfruit, passion fruit, figs, or guava. Any fresh or cooked fruit your child tolerates, cut in small bites.

Grains: Corn tortillas, brown or white rice, potatoes, yucca, yams, taro, breads, cereals, pastas, noodles, lentils, beans, quinoa, corn, and hominy.

Proteins: Lean meats including beef, pork, chicken, fish, eggs, tofu, shellfish.*

SAMPLE MENU FOR CHILDREN AGES FOUR AND FIVE

	Group	Serving	Food
Breakfast	Dairy	½ cup	4 ounces 1% milk
	Grains	1 unit	1 slice whole wheat bread
	Fat/	1 teaspoon	1 teaspoon peanut butter
	Protein Meat (optional)	1 unit	1 boiled egg
Mid-morning snack	Fruit	½ cup	4 ounces cubed cantaloupe
	Grains	½ cup	4 ounces Cheerios
Lunch	Meat	2 ounces	Baked chicken
	Vegetables	½ cup	4 ounces cubed tomatoes and cucumbers
	Fats	½–1 teaspoon	½ teaspoon low-fat salad dressing
	Grains	½ unit	½ baked potato with ketchup
	Dairy	1 cup	8 ounces low-fat flavored milk

---

*The American Academy of Allergies, Asthma and Immunology recommends waiting to introduce shellfish to children until age three.

	Group	Serving	Food
Snack	Fruit	1 cup	8 ounces natural pineapple juice
	Fat	1 ounce	2 teaspoons sunflower seeds
Dinner	Meat	2 ounces	Well-drained fried fish
	Vegetables	½ cup	4 ounces cooked mixed vegetables
	Grains	1 unit	1 small roll (optional) 4 ounces white or brown rice
	Dairy	½ cup	4–8 ounces low-fat yogurt
	Fruit	½–1 unit	1 sliced banana with the yogurt

At first glance the amount of foods might appear to be excessive; however, this sample menu includes the appropriate servings for all food groups, distributed throughout the day. Let your child decide how much he needs to eat. Refer to the Appendix for the daily calorie recommendations according to physical activity.

Despite the fact that your child can eat practically any food with any texture and size at this age, you still need to watch him to avoid choking.

The Obese Child Between the Ages of Four and Five

Most children who come to my office are sent by their pediatricians, not because their parents bring them. That's because Latino parents don't think their obese children are overweight but instead consider them to be children "who are growing up big and strong," "who look really healthy," or "who are so chubby and cute." Also, obese preschool children may not yet have experienced the jokes and teasing they're likely to suffer as they grow older.

However, if your pediatrician or dietician tells you your child is overweight, now is the time to do something about it. What you do when the child is between the ages of four and five will be so much more effective than waiting to deal with the problem later. Having said that, it's never too late to take up healthy eating and living habits.

If your children have been diagnosed as overweight or obese, *never* put them on a diet. Four- to five-year-old children are in an important stage of development and limiting what they eat can stunt their growth. Your strategy as a parent should be based on two ideas:

- Children don't need to get thinner, they only need to maintain their weight. A growth spurt will put their weight in line with their height if they start having healthy and balanced meals.

- Changing your children's food habits and preferences is something that takes time. Don't make drastic changes, just be consistent with the changes you do make. Obesity doesn't disappear overnight, but with perseverance you will notice a difference.

When you make these changes at a young age, the chances for future success in battling obesity are great. Here are some examples of what you can do to help your children think about food in a different way:

- Teach them to eat seated at the table, even if it's just a snack. Find personalized place mats, plates, and cups your children can set for themselves when they eat.

- Set the example that one shouldn't eat in front of the television. If your children get hungry, they should go to the table to eat. People eat so much more while watching television. As if that weren't bad enough, we all know food commercials only make us hungry for sweets and other foods.

- Slowly and subtly remove high-calorie low-nutrition foods and replace them with low-fat natural foods. For example, instead of buttered popcorn, try popcorn without butter; instead of doughnuts, try muffins or whole wheat rolls; or instead of ice cream, try fruit yogurt.

- Your child is now interested in knowing the why behind everything. Talk to her about why it's better to eat fresh carrots than french fries and why yogurt is better than ice cream. When children understand the different nutritional values of different foods, they'll be better able to make the right decisions about what to eat in the future.

- Take your children with you to the grocery store and let them pick out which fruits to eat or the dressing he will use to eat his broccoli or spinach. Explain how foods are arranged in different sections throughout the store and how each food group is beneficial.

- Compliment your children when they make a good choice about what to eat and explain why it's the right one. Children this age love to please their parents.

None of this means children shouldn't ever eat sweets at home. But what your child should clearly understand is that your family's first choice is healthy foods; on occasion, the sweet stuff will be fine.

Above all, remember to focus on the big picture. The idea isn't to celebrate your children not eating ice cream or cookies today, but that they've learned a positive attitude about food and how to make an educated choice about what's healthy to eat. These behavior changes will benefit them in the long run.

Parents' Attitudes Toward
Obese Children

Just as your children need to change their attitude toward food, parents and other adult relatives also need to watch how they behave toward an obese child. As I explained before, eating habits are learned. Perhaps your child has a genetic predisposition toward obesity. Still, it could be other behaviors in the household that are really causing the problem. For example:

- If there's one overweight member of the family, don't treat that person differently. Treat all members of the family the same; all of you should be eating healthy foods.

- Learn about nutrition. Chapters Three and Four explain how our bodies work and why certain nutrients are essential for good health.

- Teach your children how to eat healthy foods. Nutrition must be taught just as other household activities are: make the bed, don't pull the dog's tail, brush your teeth. No one's born knowing about nutrition.

- Don't do anything in front of your children you wouldn't want them to do: don't eat in front of the television; don't eat candy, sweets, or potato chips. If you want to eat these foods, do it sparingly and not in their presence.

- Don't buy foods you don't want your children to eat. Avoid temptations. It'll be much easier for your children to choose yogurt or fruit as a snack if they don't have to pick them over potato chips or ice cream.

And be patient. Changes in eating habits don't happen overnight. This is a learning process that takes time, just like learning to take a bath or get dressed on one's own. I always ask the parents of my patients to imagine how they picture their children as teenagers. "Do you want to see your child as a person who is capable of choosing healthy foods over bad ones and who isn't overweight? If that's your dream, then you've got to lay a foundation now that will allow your child to be that person later."

Physical Activity

Physical activity is one of the best weapons to fight and prevent obesity. Generally, children this age are very active on their own. This is when they're discovering all the interesting things the world has to offer. They rarely stop for a minute, and usually neither can you. It's not really necessary to sign up for a children's gym membership, but you should take your children outside to do fun things. Go for a walk. Play ball. This will help your children learn exercise can be enjoyable.

Your child learns by imitating what you do. If the family likes to exercise and play sports, children will learn to do that as well. If you're more sedentary and prefer watching television or other activities inside the house, then you can surely expect your children to tend to want to do those same things, also. It's really hard for adults to change their ways; but children don't have any habits until they've learned them from you. On top of this, if your child is overweight, exercising is a critical factor to maintain her weight until the next growth spurt.

A passion for physical activity is one of the best habits you can instill in your children. Exercise prevents so many of the health problems we Latinos are susceptible to, from diabetes to heart disease. This is the best age to change behaviors.

A family walk before or after dinner is an excellent form of exercise for your children and for you. Other physical activities appropriate for children this age include:

- Kicking and running after balls, big and small.

- Jumping from the first or second step on a staircase.

- Pushing a cart full of objects from one place to another.

- Climbing in safe places. Jungle gyms at the park are perfect for this.

- Walking along a line you've drawn on the floor. This will help your child develop balance.

- Playing pitch and catch with a ball. This will improve coordination.

- Dressing up in different clothes. Children this age love to become firemen, ballerinas, astronauts, or princesses. That's hard work!

- Playing Latino music. We all know how salsa makes us want to dance.

As you can see, it's not really necessary to spend money to keep a child active. It's really just a question of using your imagination.

The National Association of Sport and Physical Education (NASPE) recommends children this age have thirty to sixty minutes of organized exercise a day, as well as several hours of unstructured physical activity. In the Resource Guide you'll find contact information for this and other organizations that give advice on exercise for children.

8

Nutrition from Ages Six to Eleven

About the time your child turns six, he is entering an age of great changes. From age six until the end of his eleventh year, a child grows between one and two feet in height, and nearly doubles his weight. By the end of this period he will have become pre-pubescent, a stage when new and important changes will take place.

As far as eating is concerned, this is a time when a child's appetite generally increases considerably. The majority of my clients make the first appointments for their children around this age. Once about six years old, an overweight child is suddenly not seen as so *lindo*, or cute, anymore. The child no longer looks like the well-bred *gordito* he was at two, three, or four years old. Furthermore, it tends to be at about this age when an overweight child starts being teased by his school-mates.

There are two factors, according to a number of studies, that con-tribute to obesity in children at this age, especially in Latino children: excessive soda drinking and too many hours sitting in front of the television. These are the years when your child begins to become independent and it is important to set limits on certain behaviors, without turning it into a battle. At the same time, you'll want to give your children all the information you can on their best options when it comes to meals. Your child is reaching an age when he can better understand the concept of healthy nutrition. At least at the beginning of this stage, your child is your strongest ally in his education or reeducation regarding nutrition and physical activity: This is the stage in which children love gathering information and setting goals.

In this sense you'll need to use a bit of psychology, because the idea of a certain food "*es buena para ti,* being good for you" doesn't hold much water with children. The main influences to make them decide to choose one food over another are:

- *Taste.* Children choose certain foods because they like the taste and because those foods make them feel good.

- *Family influences.* Whatever is eaten in the home and how it is eaten is one of the greatest determining factors in your child's tastes for one food or another.

- *Friends' preferences.* At this age, friends play a very important role in the life of a child. To dress like their friends, to play the same games or eat the same foods makes a child feel like part of the group.

- *Educational programs on nutrition at school.* This information is very beneficial when it comes time for making decisions on what to eat. However, it is important that whatever they are teaching in class is also reflected in the school cafeteria so that children can choose the healthy foods they just learned about.

- *Television commercials.* Foods and restaurants that are advertised on television are also an important factor in determining a child's tastes.

This is very definitely another stage that presents new challenges and satisfactions where you, as a parent, have a great deal of influence over defining your child's tastes, as well as on his attitudes toward food and his physical activity.

From Six to Eight: A Period of Change

Six is an age when formal schooling begins and it is also the age when your child is beginning to see the world in a different way. Up until now your child has felt like the center of the universe. From now on, she will start to understand that there are other things outside of her personal universe, and her parents, family, and *amiguitos*, friends, may just have interests or feelings that are different from hers. There are also physical changes: Her baby teeth begin to fall out, her six-year-old molars come in, and there are new impulses toward her development coming from her nervous system. A typical trait at this age is that children enjoy an established routine, like knowing they will see the same teacher every day, or that their playtime and work time will come at the same time every day, and that their life at home in the evening will have a certain order of chores to be done. If your child has a routine, it will give him a feeling of security. That is why this is a good time, if you haven't done it before, to set rules for eating and schedule mealtimes. When your child is eight years old you can even post these rules, schedules, or his required chores on a board on the wall. This will help him to remember them, and to comply with them.

This is an age when children usually have good appetites, and it is normal for their "eyes to be bigger than their stomachs," or to ask for larger servings than they can possibly eat. Their tastes are very defined; whatever they like, they "love," and whatever they don't like, they "hate." Don't despair but just keep offering them healthy food, even if they refuse it time and time again.

I remember when my youngest daughter, Cassandra, was that age.

It took months for me to get her to try any dish other than white rice with soy sauce when we went out to eat in any restaurant. After having asked her dozens of times if she wanted to order some vegetables or any other healthy dish, she finally decided to do it on her own one day . . . and from that very day, she would eat absolutely anything! In any case, you also should know that it is not until the age of seven that their refusal of any new food begins to subside, and they even begin to eat things that they "don't like very much."

During this stage their table manners begin to improve, but because they are always moving, it is normal for them to bounce their legs while they're eating, so any table companion may just get involuntarily kicked a few times during the meal. Eating barefoot at home may be the easiest solution instead of trying to keep them still during meals, because very often it is simply something they cannot avoid. Talking with their mouths full is also normal, just as it is normal for them to forget two minutes later that you have just told them not to talk with their mouths full. Eating as fast as possible is also part of the program and they will frequently finish before anyone else.

Punishing a child by making him eat alone makes him feel really bad because this is an age when he is very sensitive about his failures. Although sometimes eating with small children in the family tries your patience as parents, the benefits to your child make it worth the trouble. According to one study, children who eat at the table with their families eat a better diet than those who don't; they eat more fruits and vegetables and far fewer saturated fats.

Also, toward the end of this stage, when your child is about to turn nine, she will probably be able to manage her silverware and napkins, and despite the fact that she wants to finish eating quickly to run outside and play, eating at the table with the family will be a better experience for the whole family.

TO START OFF THE DAY: *¡UN BUEN DESAYUNO!* A GOOD BREAKFAST!

Although it may seem a little ironic for a book about the obesity in Latino children, one of the biggest problems is precisely that they don't eat enough in the morning. Many Latino children don't eat a healthy breakfast and many others have no breakfast at all. The importance of breakfast for children goes far beyond a balanced diet: It is fully demonstrated that children who eat a good breakfast do far better in school.

These discoveries make sense because breakfast is the meal that gives us energy and nutrition the whole morning, and has to last until the lunch hour. When children don't eat breakfast, or don't eat a proper breakfast:

- They don't have the energy they need to function at their best.

- They don't get enough of the vitamins and minerals necessary for development. At this age children are growing, and in order to develop properly, they need a certain amount of important minerals such as calcium.

- There are studies that show that children who have breakfast at home or at school every morning have more diversity and quality in their diets than children who do not. (Also, children who participate in the School Breakfast Program consume more vitamins and minerals than those children who have a poor breakfast at home.)

- Without breakfast, they are usually so hungry by lunchtime that they eat far more and much faster than they would had they eaten breakfast.

- No breakfast means they generally go for twelve or more hours without eating, considering that the last meal they had was the day before and that the next meal they have will be lunch.

A proper breakfast for a child of this age should include:

- *Fruit or natural fruit juice.* For example, ½ to ¾ cup of fresh orange juice or a medium piece of fruit. It is much better to give them natural fruit juices instead of artificial, sweetened ones.

- *Dairy products.* Your child needs the calcium that dairy products contain for their bones and teeth to continue growing and strengthening. Dairy products include a glass of milk (8 ounces), a serving of yogurt (6 to 8 ounces), or a piece of cheese (1 to 1½ ounces).

- *Grains, breads, or cereals.* Cereals (¾ cup) should contain the smallest amount of sugar possible. You will know which is best by studying the labels. In the supermarket, search for the cereals that contain at least 2 to 3 grams of fiber per serving, although the ideal amount is 4 grams or more per serving. If your child doesn't like cereals (yet) that are a good source of fiber, don't give up but continue to offer them. There are many delicious and healthy options in cereals that children like that also offer a good balance between fiber and sugar. They can also eat a serving of toasted bread (if it is whole wheat, even better) or even a pancake with butter and jelly.

- *Proteins and/or healthy fats.* To that toasted bread, you can always add a boiled egg, a slice of low-fat ham, or peanut butter (1 to 1½ tablespoons).

This breakfast has foods from a number of food groups; try to give your child food from at least three of them. If he only eats items from two food groups at home, give him something from the third group to take with him to eat on the way to school. Believe me, just getting your child to leave the house every day with a good breakfast under his belt is a giant step toward forming healthy eating habits. Your child will have all the nutrition he needs to work properly during the school day and to cover his developmental needs.

School Breakfast Program and National School Lunch Program

These are federal meals programs available in public and nonprofit private schools. Schools that choose to participate in the programs receive cash subsidies from the U.S. Department of Agriculture for each meal they serve. In exchange, they must serve meals that meet the Dietary Guidelines for Americans, and they must offer these meals either free or for a small charge to children who are eligible.

Any child at a participating school may buy breakfast through this program, but children from families with incomes at or below 130 percent of the federal poverty level qualify for free meals. Those with incomes between 130 and 185 percent of the poverty level can buy reduced-price meals. Children from families with incomes over 185 percent of poverty pay full price. These programs provide meals every day for 27 million children in the United States.

To give you an idea, in the year 2004–2005, 130 percent of the poverty level was an income of $24,505 a year for a family of four and 185 percent was $34,873. In the Resource Guide you will find how to apply, or you can ask for more information at your child's school.

School Lunches

It is possible that during your child's day care stage you never had to face the dilemma as to whether a packed lunch from home was better than the food offered at school, but you will probably have to do it now. The first step toward making a decision whether to send your child's lunch from home or for her to eat at school is taking a good look at the menu that they offer at school. As mentioned before, if your child's school participates in the National School Lunch Program, then lunches must follow the Dietary Guidelines for Americans.

Some of the requirements set forth in the Nutritional Guidelines for Americans are to:

- Add more vegetables, fruit, and whole grains to school menus.

- Create more balanced meals by selecting foods from each of the following five food groups (grains, vegetables, fruit, dairy products, and meat or vegetable proteins).

- Reduce the fat content of meals by using less fatty meats and by offering more vegetables as main dishes.

- Serve less fried food.

- Introduce more ethnic dishes to increase variety.

In view of the current problem of childhood obesity there are many schools that offer salad and fruit bars to encourage children to eat more of these foods, even though they don't actually participate in this program. It is important to find out what options your child will have, now that he is going to have more freedom of choice. This is why it is important for him to be accustomed to eating vegetables and fruit. According to another study, children who have the option of choosing what they are going to eat at school eat less fruit and fewer vegetables and juices than those who do not have as many choices because they are served a predetermined menu.

Whichever the case may be, you can always supplement the school menu with what you serve at home. If on Fridays, for example, they serve pizza and soda, serve a dinner that includes vegetables, fruit, lean meats, and whole grains.

You may already have formed your own opinion about the breakfasts or lunches served at schools in the United States, but whatever your opinion, keep in mind that to offer a menu that satisfies children and parents from so many different cultures and culinary traditions is a true challenge for the school system. And although they may not offer very healthy foods in some schools (like the items sold in vending machines and/or through chain restaurants) it is still primarily the parents' responsibility to see that our children are provided with good nutrition.

If your child takes a lunch from home:

- Include selections from all the food groups and especially finger foods like cubes of fruit or vegetables, or nuts, because these are easier to eat.

- Maintain servings suitable for the age of your child.

- Do not send food that requires refrigeration, cooking, or reheating if the school doesn't have a refrigerator or microwave. Use an insulated lunch box so that food will stay cold or hot longer.

The following are some easy and nutritious options for school lunches:

1. Chicken wrap:
   - cold chicken strips in whole wheat wrap
   - lettuce and tomato
   - ranch-style dressing
   canned peaches

2. Ham salad:
   - cubed low-fat luncheon ham
   - lettuce and tomato
   - shredded cheese and croutons
   pear

3. Cheese quesadillas (hot):
   - soft-shell taco with shredded cheddar and Jack cheese
   - lettuce and tomato
   fresh fruit

4. Yogurt fruit dip
   - vanilla yogurt
   - sliced apples and pears, strawberries
   granola bar
   hard-boiled egg

5. Tuna sandwich
   - ▪ tuna on two slices of bread with low-fat mayonnaise
   carrot and celery sticks
   applesauce

Make your own combinations:

- ▪ a stick of string cheese
- ▪ a few crackers
- ▪ a few sections of a peeled orange
- ▪ a small cluster of grapes
- ▪ two or three peanut butter cracker sandwiches
- ▪ a small box of raisins
- ▪ a couple of celery sticks filled with peanut butter
- ▪ half a bagel with low-fat cream cheese
- ▪ small cup of cottage cheese
- ▪ small container of dry cereal
- ▪ small container of yogurt or low-fat pudding

WORK AND LACK OF PARENTAL TIME

You probably think that all the recommendations you have read on these pages are good ones, but if you are a working mother or father with a full-time job, you may be asking yourself: "Where am I going to get the time to prepare all these healthy meals?" Or, "How are we going to have family meals if each of us is on a different schedule?" Or even, "How am I going to exercise with my child in the afternoon if I never even have time enough to do my housework when I get home from work?"

Long working hours and lack of time to spend with children is a reality for millions of Latino families. At six in the evening, when many parents get home, they only have three or four hours left to organize the house, prepare and have dinner, clean up, perhaps do homework

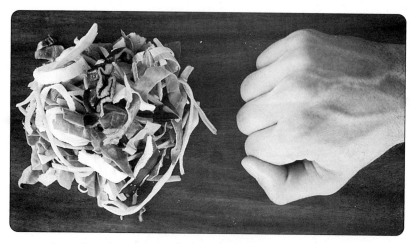

A serving of mixed vegetables should be the size of your fist.

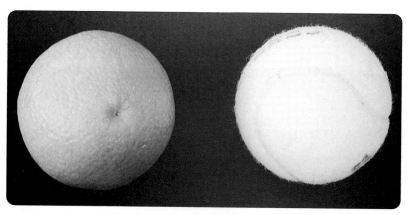

A medium-sized orange is the size of a tennis ball.

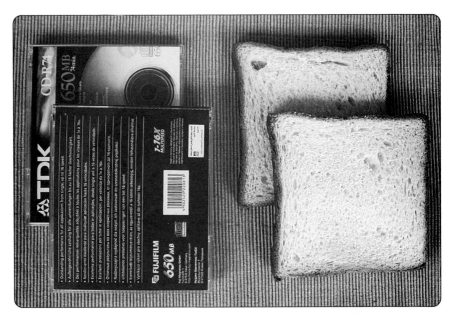

Two slices of bread should be the size of two CD cases.

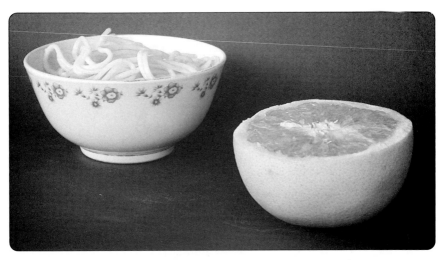

A cup of pasta is the size of a halved grapefruit.

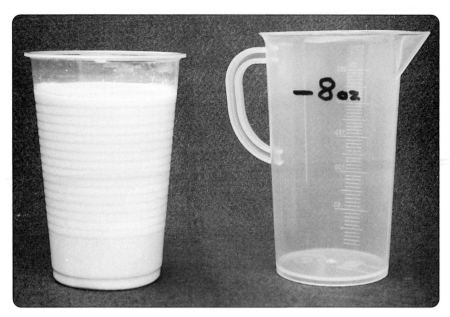

8 oz. of milk.

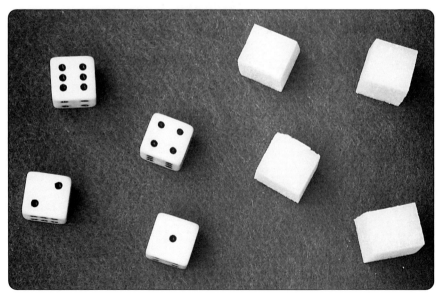

Four cubes of cheese (1–2 oz.) should be the size of four dice.

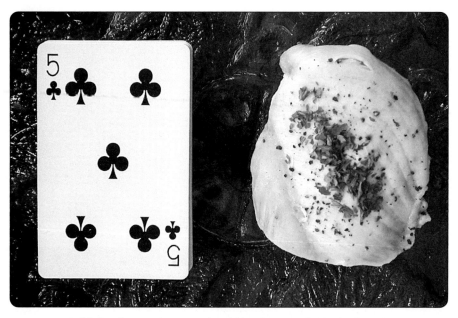

A chicken breast (3–4 oz.) should be the size of a deck of cards.

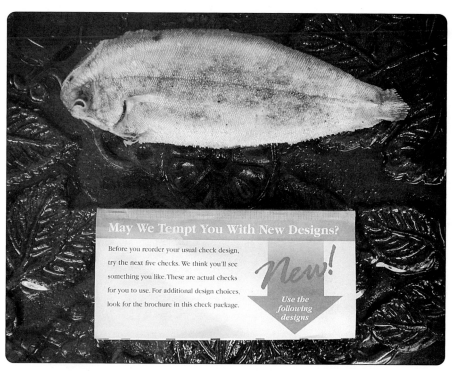

A serving of fish (3–4 oz.) should be the size of a checkbook.

1 oz. of nuts should fit in your hand.

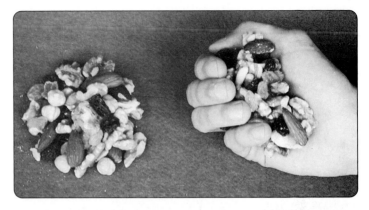

Two tablespoons of peanut butter equals the size of a Ping-Pong ball.

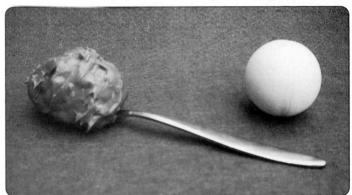

1 oz. of avocado is about the size of a highlighter.

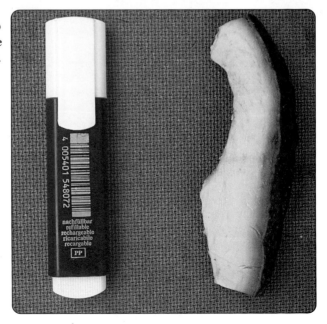

with the children, and then get everything ready for the next day. For many parents, the idea of cooking or preparing meals that take time, no matter how healthy they may be, is simply not an option. So they often end up buying prepared meals to take home or just eating in the nearest restaurant where they don't even have to wash dishes after dinner. Then with a little luck, there will still be time to watch a little television together before going to bed.

> When I was working part-time I was able to cook dinner almost every day. Now, with a full-time schedule, and working overtime often it is very difficult. Many days I just pick up some take-out dinner. Others, when I am so tired I can't even set the table, we go to a restaurant.
> —Theresa, thirty-five years old

This "fast" style of eating may work for some families, especially if they follow certain rules, like not abusing greasy foods, or eating more vegetables, or making sure that serving portions are right for the child's age. But unfortunately, in many other families this is not the case, and in the long run they will end up with problems of obesity or poor nutrition.

Making dietary changes can seem complicated and difficult to put into practice. In reality, things are easier than they seem and I can tell you, as a mother of three children with a very busy schedule, that it is possible to have a professional life and a healthy family at the same time. The whole secret is in planning.

You will find that many of the sample menus can be prepared in advance, then frozen and kept ready to serve. You can also prepare menus by buying meats that come lightly seasoned, or fruit and prewashed vegetables that are easy to serve. Following is some good advice for keeping healthy foods around without killing yourself:

- Plan your children's meals during a one- or two-week cycle and paste it on the refrigerator door.

- Just do half of the cooking: Make a list dividing fresh foods, ready to serve, like raw vegetables, from other foods that you'll be using to cook dishes (i.e., potatoes, squash, meats, fish, etc.).

- Every two weeks, or even once a month (depending on the size of your freezer), cook large amounts of the dishes that you plan to give your child or family. Then separate them into servings that are age appropriate and freeze them in clear bags, where you can see what they are, or better yet, put a label on them with the content and date the food was prepared before freezing them.

- Every night, take out the frozen servings that your child will eat the next day, and let them defrost inside the refrigerator. The next morning, or evening, you will only need to reheat the meal.

- Always have an imaginary dish in your mind in which you can switch a high-calorie meal for one with lower calories. For example, if you choose to eat fried chicken as your high calorie meal, control the serving size and fill the rest of your plate with vegetables; or if you want to serve some dessert at any given meal, don't serve bread or just serve half of the carbohydrates you ordinarily would have served. It is a question of balancing high calories with low calories on your plate.

- Have servings of raw vegetables ready to pack in your child's lunch box the next day, so that you only have to fix whatever is absolutely necessary that day. This will save you time.

If you can't have dinner together every night, at least set a few days when you can eat dinner as a family. If there are days when you have no other alternative but to dine out, then use your best nutrition judgment and all the information this book has given you to order the healthiest way possible.

- Keep in mind that servings should be sized according to age. Restaurant portions are not often normal ones, either for adults or children. Some of the biggest mistakes we make in restaurants is to order "more food for less money," or "all you can eat."

- Share an entrée with your children or take part of it home.

- Read the menu carefully and ask questions about how the meal is cooked. Try to order foods baked, broiled, grilled, poached, roasted, steamed, or sautéed and be careful with the sauces and dressings; generally they are high in calories.

- Don't be afraid to ask the waiter to "customize" your children's orders. Ask for one entrée on two plates, smaller cups for them, or for the food to be prepared in a certain way.

- For many of us who were taught to finish all our food, it's very difficult to leave food on our restaurant plates. Even when we are full, we tend to eat everything because we have paid for it. But in the end, the damage we do by eating more than we need is far more serious than any money we may have saved.

Follow the same strategy for planning a walk after dinner, or other outdoor activities. Set aside a few days to do this, even if it can only be on weekends, until you can schedule more frequent outdoor activities.

Most definitely, to teach your children and provide them with the kind of future you want for them, you have to make decisions as to where to send them to school, what activities you'll encourage, and in which social circles you want them to move. Their nutrition is no different. Children are not born knowing about healthy choices in food, so they also need to be taught in this area. If you want your child to be a healthy adult who knows what she is eating, the safest route is to begin working with her now.

I often see parents in my office who aren't familiar with the school lunch menu and don't know where to find it, either because of their difficulty with the English language or because they don't have time. One of the best practices is to sit with your child to discuss the week's menu or just the following day's menu. These school menus normally offer more than a couple alternatives that you can suggest as choices for your child. At then end of the day or after school, ask him what he ate and praise him for making the right choices. If your child didn't make the right choices that day, don't criticize him; talk to him about the other options that were available to him, without making him feel *culpable,* or guilty, by insisting too strenuously.

Menu for Children
Ages Six to Eight

Fiber is an essential element for your child in this stage of his life. Beyond being a good ally for weight control, eating foods with fiber is one of the healthiest eating habits he can learn. Foods that contain fiber are generally low in calories and provide other nutritional advantages, as is the case of grains, fruits, and vegetables.

A simple way to calculate how much fiber your child needs is to add five grams of fibers to his age. For example, if your child is six years old, you add five to his age and come up with eleven grams of fiber per day. So following this formula, a child at age eight will need approximately thirteen grams of fiber per day (8 + 5 = 13). On the nutritional information labels on food products you'll find the grams of fiber they contain. Following are examples of the fiber content of some foods:

1 medium banana	2 grams
2 slices 100 percent whole wheat bread	4 grams
1 medium orange	3 grams
3 medium-size potato wedges with skin	2 grams
½ cup peas	2 grams
Total	**13 grams**

DAILY SERVINGS FOR
CHILDREN AGES SIX TO EIGHT
Calories: 1,500 to 1,600, divided in the following way:

Food groups	Amount
Grains, legumes	2½–3 cups/units
Vegetables	2 cups or more
Fruit	2–2½ cups/units
Low-fat dairy	3 cups
Lean protein	4–6 ounces
Healthy fats	1½–2 tablespoons

Chapter Four contains some examples of recommended foods from each group. Keep in mind that at this age you should teach your child to eat fruit as it comes, that is, washed well, but with the skin on, in its original size, and without having to cut it up. The idea is that your child enjoy fruit in its natural form since you won't always be by his side to help him. Also, he can eat any raw or cooked vegetable the family eats, in small bites.

SAMPLE MENU FOR
CHILDREN AGES SIX TO EIGHT

	Group	Serving	Food
Breakfast	Protein	1 unit	1 scrambled egg
	Grain	1 slice	1 slice whole wheat toast
	Fat	½ teaspoon	½ teaspoon vegetable oil to fry
	Dairy	1 cup	8 ounces flavored low-fat (strawberry) milk

	Group	Serving	Food
Snack	Fruit	1 cup	8 ounces black grapes
	Dairy	¾–1 cup	6–8 ounces low-fat yogurt
Lunch	Grain	1–2 units	1–2 corn tortillas (6 inches each)
	Protein	2 ounces	Low-fat ground beef
	Vegetable	½–1 cup	4–8 ounces tomato, onion, and chile
	Dairy	1.5–2 oz	3 tablespoons white cheese, shredded or cubed
	Fat	½ teaspoon	½ teaspoon low-fat sour cream
Snack	Vegetable	½ cup	4 ounces celery (medium pieces)
	Fat	1 tablespoon	1 tablespoon peanut butter, spread over the celery
Dinner	Grain	½ cup	4 ounces white or brown rice
	Grain	½ cup	4 ounces black beans
	Protein	2 ounces	chicken thigh without skin
	Vegetable	1 cup	8 ounces mixed vegetables (dark greens, yellow, red) seasoned with lime, salt, and pepper to taste
	Fruit	¾–1 cup	6–8 ounces mango juice

At first glance the amount of foods might appear to be excessive; however, this sample menu includes the appropriate servings for all food groups, distributed throughout the day. Let your child decide how much he needs to eat. Refer to the Appendix for the daily calorie recommendations according to physical activity.

From Nine to the End of Eleven: The Intermediate Age

Children at this age are no longer children, but they are not adolescents either. Around the age of ten or eleven there are some physical changes, which mark the beginning of puberty. There is also a quick growth spurt, which may explain the voracious appetite of children toward the end of this stage, especially boys.

However at age nine a child's appetite begins to diminish a bit compared to the last stage from ages six to eight. Generally, they tend to stop eating quite as fast as before and they begin to take more notice of taste and texture. It is a good time to introduce foods that they haven't really liked very much until now, like fruit, which they will begin to appreciate more.

I'd never thought I'd see the day where Emma ate a whole piece of fruit without fussing. I guess all the years of insisting that she eat fruit have finally paid off!

—Faustina, forty years old

During this stage their table manners begin to improve, and they will seldom eat with their hands as they did before. All the energy that they seemed unable to control in earlier years seems to be waning, and with the exception of an occasional elbow in the ribs of whomever is closest to them, everything runs pretty well; they may even have stopped talking with their mouths full.

When they reach age ten, their appetite increases, and this includes even those children who have never eaten a lot. Potatoes tend to be one of their favorites and the vegetables they tolerate the best are green beans, although of course there are exceptions. As before, they exaggerate when expressing their food preferences; they either "adore" a food or "it makes them sick." There is no neutral term.

Around the end of their eleventh year they tend to change their preferences and what they used to like now they don't, and vice versa. This is a period in which they change their opinions and tastes often, so it's best not to give it too much importance. However, when they do like something, they can eat tremendous amounts. At eleven they can relate well to the fact that eating a lot, or eating unhealthy foods, causes them to gain weight. Precisely for this reason, it is a stage when some of them will start "diets" on their own. It is important to pay attention to the relationship that your child develops with food during this stage (see Chapter 10).

SOFT DRINKS AND CHILDREN'S OBESITY

According to national polls on nutrition, currently children between the ages of six and seventeen drink twice as much soda as before—an average of twelve ounces per day (a cup and a half), compared to the five ounces they drank daily in the 1970s. And Latino children drink more soda than any other group in this country.

This explosion in the consumption of sodas presents us with two problems. On one hand, soda and other soft drinks increase children's obesity, according to a number of studies. The calories that children drink in soda are not deducted from other foods they consume, as occurs, for instance, when they eat a lot at lunch and instinctively compensate for the excess by eating less at supper. This is because sodas are liquid and the body doesn't recognize the calories the same as it would in solid calories. So children continue to eat the same amount. A study done on the consumption of soda by children between the ages of nine and fourteen showed that those who drank nine ounces or more of soda per day added 200 more calories to their diet than the children who didn't drink sodas. Taking into account that a soda doesn't belong to any food group recommended in the pyramid, a child who drinks one can of soda a day is adding 1,400 calories per week to his diet. If that child doesn't lead an active life, these calories can turn into one or more pounds of body weight gained per month.

The other part of the problem with drinking excessive amounts of soda is that children may stop drinking milk and natural juices. This was shown in a study that followed the habits of schoolchildren for two years. In general, children who drank the most soda, in addition to the fact that they ran more risk of becoming overweight, only got three-fourths of the calcium that children who didn't drink so much soda were getting. There is research that links teenage fractures to soda and colas above all others. So in addition to losing the calcium they need, they also get far fewer vitamins A and D.

Finally, an added problem regarding drinking sweetened soda is a marked increase in tooth decay. Children who drink more soda between the ages of two and five have a much higher risk of tooth decay by the time they are seven, according to research. Latino children drink more soda than any other group in the country, and are also shown to have more tooth decay.

The American Academy of Pediatrics has recently expressed concern over the effects that these drinks have on children's health, and their availability in schools. But besides school, one of the other places where children tend to drink the most soda is while watching television at home.

What can you do to keep your child from craving soda or to reduce the amount they drink in case they already crave them? One of the most effective ways is to lead them by example. In those homes where parents drink more soda, children are three times more likely to drink soda five or more times per week. The most effective way to keep them from drinking soda at home is for you not to have it in the house, regardless of whether they are regular or diet types. It may seem like a pretty radical measure, especially if you drink a lot of soda in your house, but believe me when I say that there are other delicious and healthy drinks. When I go out with my children to a restaurant, before we go in I tell them that on this particular day they can choose "water" or "water" to drink. They are used to this and they accept it gladly because they know that there are other times when I let them drink soda.

At this age your children can understand why soda isn't good for them. Show them the amount of sugar that one soda has (10 to 12 teaspoons), or a quarter of a cup. Offer them some alternatives to quench their thirst like our traditional *aguas frescas mexicanas* (natural fruit juices diluted in water), or 100 percent natural fruit juices or flavored water with fewer than 25 calories per serving.

Just like other *dulces,* or sweets, there is no reason to eliminate all sodas from your children's diets, but you should serve them in moderation and only on special occasions.

TELEVISION, VIDEO GAMES, AND THEIR EFFECTS

When our parents were children (or even some of us), television wasn't as common in American homes as it is now. When children came home from school, they would normally go out to play in the neighborhood until it was time to come in for dinner. These hours of playing in the fresh air were an excellent way to burn energy and keep in shape.

But things have changed a lot for today's children, because of the presence of one television or more in all homes (found even in children's rooms). Other factors that contribute to excessive television are that parents don't want their children playing outside in certain neighborhoods, or that parents get home so late from work that their children are unsupervised for a while. You also need to take into account the fact that so many children have computers now where they can play video games or surf the Net, that they prefer playing them over going outside to play in the street or in their yards.

There are a number of studies that link the number of hours per day that a child spends in front of a television with their probable obesity in the future. One of them followed a group of children from the age of four until they were eleven. The results confirm that the more hours children spend in front of a television, the more overweight they become.

Watching television not only makes children overweight from a lack of physical activity but it is also a time during which children tend to consume more sodas and snacks, without paying attention to what they are eating. This fact has also been scientifically proven: The more soda they drink while watching television, the higher the probability that a child will be overweight. Furthermore, during the hours they watch television, children are bombarded by commercials advertising foods high in fats and sugars, at the rate of about ten ads per hour. These ads influence the kind of foods that children will eat later. More hours in front of a television mean a higher consumption of snacks or greasy foods, sweets or salty things, along with soda, and far less fruits and vegetables in a child's diet. This doesn't mean that you won't allow your children to watch TV at all, but you would probably need to limit the amount of hours they can sit in front of it.

Latino children are the ones who watch more television during the daytime than any other group of children in this country; the majority of them spend nearly three hours a day in front of the screen. Part of this problem stems from the long hours that so many Latino parents work. One out of every five Latino children, or a total of nearly 2 million Latino children, have to take care of themselves between the hours of three and six in the afternoon, because their parents haven't come home from work yet, and there aren't always after-school programs available in their communities; or if there are, they aren't always affordable for Latino parents.

If this is your case, you are probably facing a difficult situation, because depending on your child's age, if she is unsupervised she is likely to spend quite a few hours in front of the television, and may be eating unhealthy foods. A few things that will help a child in this situation are:

- Not keeping tempting foods like sweets, soda, or greasy or overly salted snacks in the house;

- Making an agreement with your child as to what programs she may watch daily and how much time she can spend playing with her video games; and

- Removing the television from her room, if she has one there. Having a television in a child's room is linked to obesity.

You can also give her age-appropriate chores to do around the house, like cleaning and vacuuming her room, folding her clothes, or washing them. Make a "chore board" and assign a chore every day. You'll be surprised at the amount of calories your child can burn in the course of a week or a month and furthermore, you will be helping to develop her sense of responsibility.

And one more thing; maybe you can reward all this behavior with a "healthy" video game. In response to the rising childhood obesity in the United States the video game industry has started to market video games designed to get children moving. In order to play and win, the child needs to physically move, jump, and stretch.

Menu for Children Ages Nine to Eleven

This is the stage when a child tends to eat more saturated fats (croissants, doughnuts, fast food, fatty meats, shortening, etc.), and the same holds true for sodas, while his consumption of fruit, vegetables, milk, and grains decreases. This is due to the fact that at this age they start eating "fast food" not only in restaurants but at school and at home too.

At this stage your child needs foods rich in calcium, iron, fiber, vitamins, and minerals. These nutrients are found in a variety of foods such as milk, yogurt, lean meats, cereals, whole grain breads, fruit, and vegetables.

Since your child understands your explanations so much better now, it is a good time to teach them how to eat healthily, even the foods they like the most. For example, you can prepare together a "healthy pizza" that consists of a thin dough, mozzarella cheese, tomato sauce, low-fat ham, mushrooms, slices of green pepper, and chopped tomato; and enjoy a shake made with skim milk and fruit.

It is also a good age for him to continue learning about Latin foods and for you to explain that "American" options are not always the healthiest choices.

DAILY SERVINGS FOR
CHILDREN AGES NINE TO ELEVEN
Calories: 1,600 to 1,800 calories divided the following way:

Food group	Amount
Grains, legumes	2½–3½ cups/units
Vegetables	2 cups or more
Fruit	2½–3 cups/units
Low-fat milk	3 cups
Lean meats	5–6 ounces
Healthy fats	2 tablespoons

You will find some examples of recommended foods from each group in Chapter Four.

SAMPLE MENU FOR CHILDREN AGES NINE TO ELEVEN

	Group	Serving	Food
Breakfast	Grain	¾–1 cup	6–8 ounces Cheerios
	Dairy	1 cup	8 ounces fat-free or 1% fat milk
	Fruit	1 unit	1 medium sliced banana
Snack	Grain	½–1 serving	2–4 graham crackers
	Dairy	1 tablespoon	1 tablespoon fruit-flavored low-fat cream cheese
Lunch	Grain	1 cup	Noodles or spaghetti with tomato sauce* (¼ vegetable cup)
	Protein	2–3 ounces	Shredded chicken without skin
	Vegetables	¾ cup	6 ounces steamed mixed vegetables
	Fat	1–2 teaspoons	1–2 teaspoon of margarine (light) spread or olive oil on top of vegetables
Snack	Fruit	½–¾ cup	4–6 ounces cubed papaya
	Dairy	1 cup	8 ounces low-fat chocolate milk

	Group	Serving	Food
Dinner	Grain	1 unit	1 medium malanga or yucca
	Protein	3 ounces	Baked fish seasoned with lemon and herbs.
	Salad:		
	Vegetables	1 cup	8 ounces spinach
	Fruit	½ cup	4 ounces canned mandarin orange
	Fat	1 ounce	1 ounce nuts
		1 tablespoon	1 tablespoon low-fat dressing

*Tomato sauce = vegetable

Spaghetti sauce = vegetable + carbohydrate + other ingredients

At first glance the amount of foods might appear to be excessive; however, this sample menu includes the appropriate servings for all food groups, distributed throughout the day. Let your child decide how much he needs to eat. Refer to the Appendix for the daily calorie recommendations according to physical activity.

The Obese Child Between Ages Six and Eleven

Your pediatrician or nutritionist may have confirmed that your child has a weight problem, or perhaps you have confirmed it by reading this book. In any case, it is important for you to know that as parents, it is possible to help your child, and although there may be *gorditos* in your family, this doesn't mean that your child is doomed to be chubby. Some of the most important facts to keep in mind with an obese child in this age group are:

- You cannot put a child this age on a diet because he is in a growth stage. A diet that doesn't have enough nutrients can damage your child's health.

- The home remedies like teas, herbal infusions, or diet pills to lose weight without medical supervision are not recommended for children. They can cause far more problems than the benefits they might provide. Something as simple as *sávila* or aloe vera can give a child diarrhea. Be very careful not to give him supplements or diet preparations for adults, even though they seem perfectly natural. Your child is going through a stage of development and these remedies can have serious side effects.

- Do not blame your child for being overweight. Your child's eating habits have a lot to do with the family's eating habits, as well as its physical activity. Children learn from what goes on around them.

- Don't demand that he do things you do not do. If you don't like vegetables, you can't insist that your child eat them. To teach him by example is the most effective weapon you have, so trying to improve your diet will help your child.

- The goal in treating an obese child is not for him to lose weight but for him to learn a series of healthy eating habits and to develop a liking for physical activity that will last him a lifetime.

- Don't give him a "nutrition plan" and expect that the child will do it on his own. Just as in so many other areas of his education, as parents you need to get directly involved with him.

- Don't expect spectacular changes either in your child's physical appearance or in his habits. There is no "magic" remedy for obesity. Changes in attitudes toward food and physical activity come about little by little. The important thing is that your child assimilate them to slowly put them in practice.

■ Education about nutrition is one of your best tools. Children between the ages of six and eleven understand the reasons why some foods are healthy and some are not. Explain what you have learned in this book in plain language that your child can understand.

■ Praise your child when he chooses a healthy food. Above and beyond nurturing his self-esteem, you will be teaching him the best choices in foods.

■ Avoid any kind of humiliating comment regarding his obesity or his physical appearance, whether you are alone with him or around other people. His self-esteem is a very delicate thing, and you can harm your child.

■ Do not compare your child to his siblings, relatives, or friends. Every individual has a distinct physical appearance and different physique from everyone else and your child is unique and special, as are all your other children.

Remember that helping your child to modify his relationship with food along with his physical activity is a task in which the entire *familia* should participate. At least at the beginning children don't know how to do it alone.

If your child has been diagnosed with a complication related to his obesity, like diabetes, high blood pressure, or high cholesterol, then you should work with his pediatrician or a nutritionist in a proper program. In Chapter Eleven you will find information about some of these conditions, and in the Resource Guide, places where you can get help and advice about nutrition.

TEASING BY SCHOOLMATES

One of the hardest parts for both the obese child and her parents is watching her suffer because of comments made by her schoolmates or because *seburlan*, they tease her. At this age friends are very important to her; her friends become the center of her universe. Whomever she sits with at lunchtime, what team she is on, or whether or not she is invited to a birthday party all become very important things that bring on many tears and sadness. Friends are necessary for the emotional development of your child and so a comment like "*Eso no es importante,* that's not important" or "You'll find new friends" doesn't tend to help much, but rather quite the opposite. And although you have probably thought about it more than a few times, it is also not a good idea to talk to all the children who tease your child. However, there are certain attitudes on your part that can help your child to overcome this situation:

- Establish good communication with her. It will help her a lot to talk about what has occurred in school and for you to listen to her. Ask her questions about the situations she encountered and show interest in everything that occurred. Talk to her about her feelings about the teasing. You don't necessarily need to give her a solution to the problem if you don't have any; just listening to her and sharing her feelings is one of the best ways you can help her.

- Make positive comments about the qualities your child has in other areas. It is important for her to feel worthwhile about things that have nothing to do with her physical appearance. For her to feel valued by her *familia* is one of the biggest boosts you can give her self-esteem.

- Schedule a meeting with your child's teacher to learn more about the situation and what kind of measures the school is taking to control this type of behavior toward obese children. Learn the teacher's opinion regarding the effect that this teasing has had on your child.

THE LATINO FAMILY AND THE OBESE CHILD

If your family lives nearby, they are a factor to be taken into account if you are making an effort to change the eating habits of your child, especially if your child spends time frequently with his *tíos*, aunts and uncles, or *primos*, cousins, or at his *abuelitos'*, grandparents', house— especially if your mother or mother-in-law takes care of him part of the day.

For many of our older family members, a *gordito*, or chubby child, is thought of as a healthy child, regardless of our pediatrician's many warnings that he can develop diabetes, high cholesterol, or any other problem related to obesity. Besides, how can one reject all those delicious dishes and desserts that *abuelita* prepares so lovingly for her grandchild?

> *It was very difficult to convince my mother-in-law that she couldn't give to Raul all the sweets and desserts he wanted. For her Raul's obesity was not a problem. Only when I took her with me to the pediatrician, she started to understand that her gordito was having health problems.*
> —María Patricia, twenty-six years old

In so many of our families, to cook for others is a symbol of love, and to refuse those dishes is even considered offensive. The best way to clear up misunderstandings is to have a talk alone with the *abuelitos* or other family members who spend time with your child to explain the situation to them and ask for their collaboration. It is important to communicate that you appreciate how wonderful these meals are and how much love and effort goes into preparing them. Make sure they understand you are not rejecting them but rather trying to avoid the child's suffering both physically and psychologically because of being overweight.

Taking your mother or mother-in-law with you to the doctor's appointment with the pediatrician or nutritionist so she can get this information firsthand and can participate more directly in her grandchild's new attitudes toward food is a good idea too, especially if she is in charge of some of your child's meals. Kindly explain to her that she shouldn't make your child *dejar el plato limpio*, finish everything on his plate, nor should she use food as a reward or punishment.

Encourage them to try out recipes for dishes that use more vegetables, lean meats, and fish. Latino cuisine has many healthy and delicious options.

HEALTHY CHANGES IN YOUR FAMILY'S NUTRITION

One of the first changes that you can put into practice in your family is replacing the phrase *"esto es engorda,* this is fattening" with *"esto es saludable,* this is healthy." The idea is to emphasize healthy food choices rather than things that make us look fat or thin. Even if this seems a little silly, it is a change that will turn the focus toward nourishment for both you and your child in a completely new way.

If there is a problem of obesity either in your family or your husband's, it is logical to be tempted to control what your child eats because they don't want him or her to "get fat" too. But research shows that you get far better results by not forcefully controlling what your children eat but rather focusing on everything regarding their meals from a "healthy" point of view. Following are some healthy options that your family can adopt to help your overweight child:

- Plan three meals a day with one or two snacks between them. If your child is hungry earlier, you don't necessarily have to give him another meal or snack, but you can shift the meal schedule up just a bit.

- Plan healthy family meals ahead of time, as this will help save time and you'll be able to avoid last-minute meals where you fix the first thing you find in the refrigerator.

- Take your child shopping with you. Let him choose his favorite vegetables and the seasoning with which he wants to eat them, but be sure these are low in fats. Also, your child may just know more than you do about one or another aspect of nutrition, because he has been studying this in school. Share in his knowledge.

- Avoid keeping things in the house that you don't want your child to eat, like potato chips, cookies, *dulces,* sweets, candy, and greasy snacks. Keep healthy alternative snacks around like fruit cut up in cubes, natural juices, or dairy products.

- Encourage your child to help in cooking healthy food. He will feel far more inclined to try things if he "helped" to cook them.

- Plan family meals without television, like in the old days. Try to make it a pleasant moment for sharing the day's experiences.

- Keep in mind what a properly sized serving is, according to your child's age.

- Serve healthy food to all members of the family. Don't make a special menu just for the person with a weight problem.

- If your overweight child is the youngest of a number of siblings, observe what he is eating. Sometimes a child will eat too quickly and excessively because he is afraid he will go hungry.

Above all, always have a big reserve of patience on hand. Children are not fond of change, but if they see that you are bound and determined to make the changes, they will eventually accept them and even collaborate with you.

Physical Activity

This is the age when children tend to spend hours sitting in front of a television or playing video games. School-age children need at least thirty minutes to one hour of physical exercise a day, and another hour just for play.

Physical activity is a family affair. Just as in many other areas, your child tends to repeat the behavior he sees at home, and if he sees that you prefer watching television most of the time over going to the park or taking a walk in the fresh air, it is very likely that your child will share the same preference. After a hard day at work, only to come home in the afternoon to fix dinner, clean, and get things ready for the next day, it is likely that the idea of going out to get some exercise with your child, even just in the yard, is just more of an effort than you can make. So the only thing you feel like doing is watching television quietly for a while. Forcing yourself to exercise with your child doesn't tend to work in the long run, because if it isn't something that you both can enjoy with the rest of the family, you simply won't do it. You need to change habits little by little toward a more active lifestyle. For example:

- Walk whenever possible, instead of driving.

- Use the stairs instead of taking the elevator.

- Walk around a shopping center, without necessarily shopping or eating.

- Organize family reunions in parks or places where the children can run and play outdoors.

- If you have a dog, walk it together.

- Teach your children to dance salsa at home and keep this kind of music playing in the background instead of the television. Latin rhythms help to keep us active!

In addition, you can't count on your child getting all the physical exercise he needs in school. Unfortunately many schools don't even offer physical activities, or they don't offer the hours that children require. This is why it's important to find a physical activity that you, your child, and the rest of the family can enjoy and practice often. This can be anything from playing football to taking salsa classes or going to a skating rink.

If you live in a neighborhood where there are other children the same age as yours, perhaps you can take turns with other mothers and fathers, and take the children to a park or let them get together in different homes to play together. Another option is to enroll them in some after-school physical activity program at school or at another community institution. However, this option is sometimes a problem for Latino parents. According to a recent study, many Latino parents cannot do this because they have transportation or financial problems, or they simply have no time, or because there aren't any activities or any type of sports or physical exercise programs for children in their area. There are other Latino parents who have a problem because of their English, either because they don't know how to look for information about these programs or because they fear they won't be able to communicate with the coach.

All of these problems are very real, but thanks to the campaigns that have been put into effect recently to help children get the exercise they need, you may just find an alternative in your community that fits your needs. The first step in learning about these programs is to look for information. In Chapter Twelve you will find the contacts that might help you.

JOIN A TEAM

Team sports, like football or basketball, are physical activities where a child this age can fit in easily. Apart from being a source of physical exercise, to belong to a team is a very positive boost for a child's self-esteem. In the special case of Latino children who are just beginning to become a part of this new culture, to be on a sports team can help them feel closer to their schoolmates.

Generally, children may begin to take part in team sports from the age of six. However, there are children this age who are not yet ready for a competitive sport where the team members are pressured, and in that case it is better to wait a little longer until the child is ten or eleven, or look for other physical activities that are more appropriate for his age.

At schools there are usually teams for different sports that your child can join. But above all, don't forget that the first requisite for things to work out is that your child have fun while he is playing.

OVERWEIGHT CHILDREN AND EXERCISE

If your child is overweight, physical exercise is one of your best options to help her burn calories, just as it is a basis for forming healthy habits. However, it is important to understand that for an overweight child, exercise may not be easy, for several reasons:

- She may become tired faster than the others, or may not be able to jump as high or run as fast as the rest.

- To avoid the other children teasing her about her physical fitness, she may refuse to exercise with other children.

- She may not want to be seen in a bathing suit or in shorts, and may refuse to go to the swimming pool or to a physical activity program with other children.

- She may not want to be a part of a team because she feels she is not as good as the other children.

- Being overweight may cause her pain in certain parts of her body, like her feet or back. If this is the case, you should consult your pediatrician immediately.

If you are living with one of these situations, try to understand your child's feelings and help her as much as possible. An overweight child needs your help and support to improve her physical condition. For example, if she feels badly about the clothes she has to wear in front of the other children to do sports, then, when you shop, let her pick the clothes that will make her feel the most comfortable.

If she doesn't want to do exercise with other children, perhaps she can do it at home with a video, take walks with you or the family, or even go swimming at a pool. Swimming is one of the best exercises for overweight children, because it doesn't place stress on the joints.

But just as important as focusing on increasing physical activity in an overweight child, you must try to reduce or eliminate activities that keep your child from being active. It is shown that just cutting the hours your child spends watching television or playing video games, in addition to taking the television out of his or her room, will automatically increase a child's physical activity.

And remember that in all the strategies you plan in order to help your child be more active, you need to be very patient and persistent. Lasting changes don't happen overnight. Furthermore, even if there are times when it seems as if you are taking two steps backward for every one you take forward, the important thing is to know you are staying on the path.

9

Nutrition from Ages Twelve to Nineteen

Adolescence is a crucial stage in life. "Perhaps it is one of the most difficult stages for us as it is for our parents, because it is a crisis that involves our entire personality. Our bodies change, we grow suddenly, our way of dressing, our sexuality and all these changes concern us and we don't understand where we stand, what we want or where we're going."

This is how a group of teenagers describes this stage on a Web site created by them to talk about adolescence. "The change" is definitely the main theme in adolescence according to my adolescent clients' parents who often are distressed by the changes. One of the leading reasons for parents coming to me is that "We cannot control what she eats," "*Ha cambiado tanto,* she has changed so much, and we don't know what to do about her eating," or "Could you talk to him and make him see reason?" These situations refer as much to adolescents who are overweight as those who have eating disorders.

The stage between the ages of twelve and nineteen denotes the main years when the greatest physical and psychological changes take place—or in other words, the stage in which children stop being children and start to become adults. With respect to nutrition and obesity, it is a very important stage for a number of reasons:

- Latino children between the ages of twelve and nineteen, as a group, are the most obese in the entire country.

- Adolescence is the last critical stage in the development of obesity as an adult, due to the changes that take place both in the amount and in the location of body fat.

- The type of obesity that develops or persists during adolescence is associated with more serious health complications.

- Obese teenagers are much more likely to become obese adults.

A lot of growth takes place during these years, which goes hand in hand with weight gain, especially in girls. For girls, the weight gain during adolescence, if excessive, can have consequences on the extent and persistence of their obesity as adults. This is due to the fact that the adipose or fat cells don't disappear when a person loses weight but simply reduce in size: the number of cells remains the same. The more adipose or fat cells that exist, the more the risk of developing obesity.

In boys, adolescence doesn't necessarily bring about a weight gain, but it does cause a redistribution of fat deposits. Fat is now distributed around the body in a different way than it was during childhood. Boys tend to accumulate fat in the abdomen much more than girls. Abdominal fat is related to what we call visceral fat and can be harmful to health. Latinos, because of hereditary factors, have a higher propensity to accumulating abdominal fat. This excess of visceral fat is related to two of the most common disorders that affect obese Latino children: resistance to insulin and metabolic syndrome.

Because of the previous risks, this is a very important stage in which to establish and reinforce some healthy nutritional habits and also to take the proper steps in case your child has a weight problem;

but always keep in mind that youngsters in this stage of development have special needs.

From Twelve to Fifteen: Puberty

Puberty is a word that refers to the physical changes that take place during these years; the word *adolescence* refers to the psychological changes that accompany the physical changes. The physical changes at this stage have the greatest effect on the sexual organs.

In girls, toward the end of age twelve on average is when menstruation begins and also when their breasts begin to develop. There are girls who are more prepared for this change than others. Communication with your daughter is very important because she may be afraid of these changes or there may be things she hasn't understood very well. Even though she's taking classes in school on the physical changes in her body, your daughter will feel more secure if she can talk about it with you. Encourage her to ask you about anything she doesn't understand. During adolescence, keeping the lines of communication open to your children is the best way to prevent behavior that can cause tension.

Regarding boys, some develop more quickly than others at this stage. This is the age when their sexual organs grow and when they begin to get hair on their legs and faces. This is also accompanied by a change in the pitch of their voices. You, and especially your husband (or a male figure) can help them avoid anxiety by talking about the changes that they are going through in a very natural way. It is as common for boys as for girls to be preoccupied by what is happening to them and to constantly compare themselves to their friends.

This entire development brings about a noticeable increase in appetite; after eating two servings of lunch, they may even complain that they are still hungry. Some children insist that they aren't hungry in the morning hours, but will devour everything in sight at lunchtime. In the afternoon, after coming home from school, the first place they head for is the kitchen, to find something to eat.

*Tony, my son, was complaining the other day about the frozen yogurt
not being frozen enough. No wonder! That door of the fridge spends
more time open than closed!*

—Samuel, forty-five years old

This huge appetite is perfectly normal for an adolescent, but precisely for this reason it is important to help him regulate it in as healthy a way as possible by starting the day out with a good breakfast, taking nutritious lunches to school, eating healthy dinners, and having healthy, quick snacks around the house. Due to this increased appetite, this is the stage when they are more open to trying foods that they haven't liked before, for instance certain vegetables or fruits.

FAST FOOD

In the last few decades, the adolescent diet has changed considerably in the United States. The number of calories that young people consume today is much higher than teenagers used to consume, and furthermore, the percentage of calories that come from fat and saturated fats is far higher now. They eat far more french fries and pizzas than they used to, they drink far more sodas and sweetened drinks, and they drink much less milk. This isn't strange since according to one study, an adolescent's favorite meals are, in this order: pizza, ice cream, spaghetti, french fries, hamburgers, puddings, cornflakes, potato chips, and popcorn.

In adolescence, friends take on a big role in a youngster's social life, and this social life often involves going to a mall, see a movie, and of course . . . eat in fast-food restaurants. For many teenagers this is part of their "culture." Although nutritionally this is not the best kind of food to eat frequently, it won't really hurt your child when eaten occasionally, as long as he or she eats healthier food the rest of the week. That is to say, now that your child has his own access to other types of food, it is important that:

■ The weekly menu contains enough vegetables, fruit, grains, and milk products for his body to have what it needs to develop during this time of great growth.

■ You try to limit, at home, any prepared foods with a lot of fat, sugar, or salt, to compensate for the meals that your child has on his own.

■ You explain to your child how important it is for his physical development to eat a balanced diet. There are a good number of studies documenting the link between fast food and malnutrition in teenagers.

■ You talk to him about other possible choices of "acceptable" foods when he goes out with his friends. It is very important for teenagers to be part of the crowd and they don't want to stand out as being different from the rest.

One of the best things you can do for the future health of your child is to educate him about nutrition. There are studies that show that when teenagers have the option of choosing their own food at school where there are food vending machines or cafeterias where they can choose things from a menu, they tend to eat fewer vegetables and fruit. Excessive teenage consumption of fast food is also related to having a job, watching a lot of television, or having this type of food too easily available at home.

HEALTHY BONES, HEALTHY TEETH: CALCIUM IN ADOLESCENTS

There is a general belief among Latinos that once childhood is over, milk is no longer needed—something like, "milk is for *bebés*." However, the teen years may be the most important stage for developing healthy bones. At the end of this period most of the body's bone structure has finished growing. Not getting enough calcium during this stage can make for serious bone problems in the future.

Investigators have detected that in Latino children, and especially in girls, there are great reductions in calcium intake at this age. One of the things to blame for this, according to other studies, are sodas and sweetened drinks. As the child grows she tends to drink less milk, while she drinks more and more sodas. By the time children reach adolescence, they are drinking twice as many sodas and sweetened drinks as milk. An added problem in drinking less milk is that they can also develop a vitamin D deficiency. Since this vitamin is added to milk, milk is its main dietary source. On the other hand, not only are bones affected by this change, but teeth too; Latino children are the group with the most cavities in the United States.

It is clear that sodas and sweetened drinks are not good for your child because they not only reduce the calcium your child gets but they increase the number of calories that your child consumes per day without increasing the amount of nutrients.

Calcium is not only found in milk. Yogurt, cheese, kale, collard greens, spinach, and canned sardines also have calcium. If your child is not a milk lover, these other foods will give him the calcium that he needs; however, dairy foods are the easiest way to get this needed mineral. For example, a glass of milk contains about 300 mg of calcium, while your child would need two cups of cooked collard greens to get the same amount. I often ask my children what sources of calcium or other nutrients they had on any given day. That doesn't mean that I am drilling them. We make it a kind of game, but they know that this is something they need to consider when they decide their own menus.

In case your child doesn't eat any food that contains calcium, you should consult his pediatrician or nutritionist about the possibility of giving him a calcium supplement, but always continue to offer him foods that are rich in this mineral. "Real" foods are the main source of nutrients, and a diet based on supplements doesn't make up for foods. Healthy bones during adolescence are the basis for healthy bones later in life.

EATING DISORDERS

At this age children, above all girls, become very conscious of their figures. This is the stage when most eating disorders develop. Given how difficult it is to treat these illnesses and the impact that they can have on your child's health, prevention is the best remedy.

Overweight Latinas suffer more of these illnesses than other girls, especially the compulsive bingeing disorder. Generally food is not the problem but rather the need to be accepted by the crowd that leads them to go on extreme diets, then binge, purge, take laxatives, and all the other behaviors that go hand in hand with eating disorders. These illnesses are dealt with in more depth in Chapter Ten.

One important thing that your daughter should know is that this type of diet, instead of helping her to lose weight, does just the opposite. According to a study that followed more than 15,000 children nine to fourteen years old, girls who diet and then binge gain more weight than those who don't diet but exercise more. Investigators believe that dieting this way makes the metabolism readjust and makes the body work with fewer calories; or in other words, these diets make the body use less energy so that everything one eats is stored in the most efficient way, as fat. However, small changes, like drinking skim milk instead of whole milk, or including a few fruits and vegetables in a diet, or doing more exercise, can achieve an adjustment in a teenager's weight.

Talk to your son or daughter about these things; explain what eating disorders are and boost their self-confidence and self-image. Low self-esteem is the root of all of these diseases.

Menu for Children Ages
Twelve to Fifteen

The calories that your son or daughter consumes at this age can vary by gender. Although both boys and girls need enough calories to keep growing, generally boys eat more than girls: between 200 and 400 more calories per day, depending on their physical activity.

By this age your child should be eating a wide variety of foods, in proper portions, and if there is something he doesn't like or it's the first time he has seen it, it is important to reason with him and not let him simply say no until he has at least tried the food. In other words it is at this age when the battles at the dinner table should have come to an end. Despite this, if he still doesn't like certain foods, whether new to him or not, it is very possible he will accept them soon. Neither you nor your child should give up.

> It is certainly a relief to see that at least she listens to me when I explain why she should try a new food. Before there was no way to reason with her. Even if she decides not to try what I am offering her, I know that some of what I am explaining about good eating habits is sticking.
>
> —Gloria, thirty-nine years old

Unquestionably, your child's favorite food will probably be a hamburger and potato chips, and it is next to impossible to fight with him about it, and sometimes unnecessary. Instead of concentrating on criticizing him or trying to make him eat only vegetables in a fast-food restaurant, try to focus on what you can do for him at home and about the information and advice that you can give him regarding his nutrition. At this point, your child is able to understand perfectly how a balanced diet is essential for his development, for energy, and for getting good grades in school. Explain patiently, and without pressuring him or getting angry at him, that if he doesn't choose healthy foods for most of his meals, he can become an obese teenager, raise his blood pressure and cholesterol levels, and can actually end up with diabetes or coronary disease at a very early age. Don't forget that practicing what you preach is the most efficient way to teach your child to eat healthily.

Some of the most necessary nutrients for this stage of growth are proteins, calcium, iron, zinc, and fiber, among others. A typical teenage diet is generally lacking in these nutrients. In Chapter Three you will find information about foods rich in them.

DAILY SERVINGS FOR
ADOLESCENTS AGES TWELVE TO FIFTEEN
Calories: 1,800 to 2,200 divided the following way:

Food group	Amount
Grains, legumes	3½–4 cups/units
Vegetables	2–2½ cups or more
Fruit	2½–3 cups/units
Low-fat dairy products	3 cups
Lean meat	6 ounces
Healthy fats	2 tablespoons

In Chapter Four you will find some examples of recommended foods from each group.

SAMPLE MENU FOR ADOLESCENTS
AGES TWELVE TO FIFTEEN

Calories may be higher or lower, depending on the physical activity of your child. A sedentary child twelve years of age can consume 1,800 calories daily, while an active child the same age can eat 2,400. The following menu is based on a diet of 2,000 calories, so there is room to increase or lower the calories depending on the amount of exercise your child gets.

	Group	Serving	Food
Breakfast	Grain	1 unit	1 medium bagel
	Dairy	1–1.5 ounces	1.5 ounces *queso blanco* or 2 tablespoons low-fat cream cheese
	Fruit	1 cup	8 ounces fresh orange juice
Snack	Vegetables	½ cup	4 ounces baby carrots and celery
	Fat	1 tablespoon	1 tablespoon low-fat ranch dressing
	Dairy	¾ to 1 cup	6–8 ounces fat-free or 1% milk
Lunch	Pizza:		
	Grain	2 units	1 *individual* piece pizza dough
	Protein	2–3 ounces	Low-fat ham over the pizza dough
	Vegetable	2 ounces	4 tablespoons tomato sauce*
		2 ounces	4 tablespoons green and red pepper and onion over pizza
	Dairy	2 ounces	4 tablespoons melted mozzarella cheese over pizza
Snack	Fruit	1 unit	1 medium pear

	Group	Serving	Food
Dinner	Salad:		
	Protein	3 ounces	Tuna in water seasoned with lemon
	Vegetable	1½ cup	8–12 ounces mixed vegetables (lettuce, tomatoes, zucchini)
	Grain	¼ cup	2–4 tablespoons low-fat croutons
	Fat	1 tablespoon	1 tablespoon low-fat salad dressing
	Fruit	½ cup	4 ounces white grape juice

*Tomato sauce = vegetable

Spaghetti sauce = vegetable + carbohydrate + others

At first glance the amounts of foods might appear to be excessive; however, this sample menu includes the appropriate servings for all food groups, distributed throughout the day. Let your child decide how much he needs to eat. Refer to the Appendix for the daily recommendations according to physical activity.

From Fifteen to Nineteen: Adolescence

During the first years of this stage, the tremendous physical changes that have taken place in the last few years finally begin to stabilize. But along with these physical changes, a lot of psychological changes have taken place too. The main personality trait in an adolescent is his need for independence, to do things for himself and to test his limits. During this process, his friends become a very important part of his life because teenagers search for their own identity in their groups of friends, and generally, or at least in this stage, their identities tend to be very different from those of their parents. To understand them, just remember your own teenage years and what you liked.

This type of relationship with friends is normal, and it would never be possible for children to become independent people without this process. Although you may have some tense situations where your child is testing his new limits, it doesn't mean that adolescence has to be a battleground; but it is a time when your parenting skills are going to be tested. The secret is to establish boundaries that are not too rigid, but have boundaries in place. Your child still needs your guidance, especially when it comes to nutrition.

Family meals at this stage, above and beyond helping your child eat properly, are a magnificent moment to talk, and to keep the lines of communication open with your teenager. Talking and listening to your teenager is the best way to find out what is going on in his life. One way to get your child to participate more in these meals is to let him cook a dinner, or cook it with him once a week, or do the shopping with him so he can help decide what you're going to serve.

TEENAGERS' APPETITES AND VENDING MACHINES

Almost every high school in the United States has one or more vending machines that sell snacks and sodas. One of the main reasons why schools accept these machines is because it brings in more revenue that can be spent on programs, material purchases, or repairs. The problem with these machines is that the great majority of the products they sell are snacks with a high fat and salt content, sweets, and sodas and other sweetened drinks. There are very few vending machines in schools that offer healthy snacks. Fortunately recent initiatives are trying to change this situation.

Now that your child probably has a little money of her own, it is hard to control what she eats from these machines, but there are a few measures you can take to prevent, or at least minimize, her using them.

■ Be sure she eats a good breakfast every morning. Plan her waking time to be sure she has time for a good breakfast. Not only will it help with her performance in school but it will help her avoid the temptation to buy unhealthy snacks if she has access to a snack and soda vending machine at school.

■ The night before, help her prepare or teach her to prepare something healthy as a midmorning snack (fruit, milk, a small serving of whole wheat), so that it's ready for her to take in the morning.

■ Talk to her about the benefits of a good diet and about the special importance of staying healthy during her adolescent years to help her avoid gaining weight in the future.

HEALTHY HABITS: HEALTHIER LIFE

Around this age there are many adolescents who already have part-time jobs, after-school activities, homework to do when they get home, and who also spend time talking on the phone, watching television, or surfing the Net.

With such busy schedules, it is common for many teenagers not to find time to sleep enough hours, follow proper hygiene, or prepare healthy meals. This situation tends to become a vicious circle: The less sleep they get, the worse their performance in school, the more tired they feel, and then the less time they have to follow a healthy diet. An unhealthy diet has another consequence too, which is for the child to feel less energy and more fatigue. Keeping reasonable hours in order to get enough rest is the first step in establishing a healthier lifestyle. Furthermore, recent studies have shown that people who sleep less produce less of the hormone that suppresses appetite, and as a result, they feel compelled to eat meals with higher calories and more carbohydrates.

Adolescents need a minimum of eight hours of sleep, or more, to feel rested the next day. Two measures you can take to see that your child sleeps enough are:

- Establish a reasonable schedule for your child's after-school activities, giving priority to sports. Remember that he needs time every day to do his homework.

- Don't install a television, an Internet connection, or a telephone in your child's room. Many parents give their children televisions, telephones, or Internet connections, but it is much too common to see adolescents spending far too many afternoon hours glued to the telephone, surfing the Internet, or watching television. Tell him that he can do this in the family room, where you will have far more control over the number of hours he spends on these activities. If he already has a computer in his room, establish a schedule that he will follow.

Personal hygiene is something that some teenagers tend to neglect. If your child doesn't have time to bathe in the mornings, encourage her to take a relaxing bath at night; beyond keeping her skin clean and helping her improve problems with acne, it will also help her relax before going to sleep. Be sure she doesn't forget to brush her teeth.

Make her diet a priority. Keep healthy snacks in the refrigerator and prepare what she'll be taking to school the night before to avoid rushing around at the last minute in the morning. If your child is rested, clean, and well fed, her performance, both at school and at work, will be better, and she'll be able to avoid the vicious circle of unhealthy behavior.

DEPRESSION IN ADOLESCENTS

For some adolescents, the changes and adjustments of this stage of life are sometimes too much, especially if they coincide with other circumstances like family problems, the death of a loved one, or, in the case of some Latino children, the loss of friendships and relatives in their homeland and adapting to a new culture. As a matter of fact, Latino adolescents have the highest rate of depression at this age, and are the ones who think the most about suicide or even attempt it, especially boys. Some of the signs of depression that could indicate a problem are:

- Depressed or irritable mood.

- Apathy, little interest in anything.

- Difficulty in sleeping or excessive sleepiness during the day.

- Loss of, or increased, appetite.

- Difficulty in concentrating.

- Irresponsible or defiant behavior.

- Suicide attempts.

If you observe one of these symptoms or believe that your child may be depressed, you should consult his doctor. There are certain illnesses, like hypothyroidism (underfunctioning of the thyroid gland), that can produce some of these symptoms. It is important to consult a professional before taking drastic steps, if you feel your child's behavior is unusual or he is involved in fights; or if you suspect he may be using drugs.

One of the most effective preventive measures is to keep the lines of communication with your adolescent open, especially if you are all adapting to a new culture or if your family is going through a crisis of some sort. Two of the places where you will have the best chance to encourage this communication is at the table during family meals, or going out to practice a sport or some other physical activity with your child.

Menu for Young Adults
Ages Sixteen to Nineteen

Your child's nutrition during adolescence will have a strong impact on his future. A nutritious diet in this stage can determine your child's health later on when it comes to his bones, muscles, heart, arteries, and immune system. In this stage, the calories your child eats daily can differ enormously from those of his school friends, depending on his growth rate, his present or final height, and his physical or sports activity. Just like adolescents ages twelve to fifteen, youngsters from sixteen to nineteen years old have shortages in proteins, calcium, iron, zinc, and fiber. These nutrients are essential throughout the entire stage of accelerated growth.

The requirement for vitamins increases at this stage too, especially the B vitamins (thiamine/B_1, riboflavin/B_2, niacin/B_3, B_6, B_{12}, and folate) that are found in whole grains, fortified cereals, animal protein, green vegetables, legumes, nuts, and seeds. Furthermore, the need for vitamins D, A, C, and E also increases. Milk, though not all other dairy products, is rich in vitamin D. Vitamin A is found in whole milk, fortified low-fat milk, liver, eggs, carrots, dark green vegetables; and vitamin C in red and green peppers, dark green vegetables, broccoli, tomatoes, potatoes, strawberries, and citrus fruit. In Chapter Three you will find ample information on all of these nutrients.

When I have an adolescent in my office, I often see parents who are very worried about nutrition or specific foods. For example, one mother served her sixteen-year-old daughter liver every day to prevent an iron-deficiency anemia; and while doing so was giving her an abundance of all kinds of foods. In her efforts to make sure her daughter got all the iron she needed, this mother was also making her overweight. In summary, the important thing is to get our children used to eating a wide variety of foods instead of focusing on one specific thing, unless this has been ordered by his or her doctor.

Have conversations with your adolescent child about whether he is eating vegetables and fresh fruit, if he is eating too many starches as most of us Latinos do, if he consumes enough milk products, and/or if your child, especially if a girl, is on a diet without you knowing it.

DAILY SERVINGS FOR
YOUNG ADULTS AGES SIXTEEN TO NINETEEN
Calories: 2,200 to 2,600 divided the following way:

Food group	Amount
Grains, legumes	4½–6 cups/units
Vegetables	2–3½ cups or more
Fruit	3½–4 cups/units
Low-fat dairy products	3 cups
Lean meat	6 ounces
Healthy fats	2 tablespoons

In Chapter Four you will find some examples of recommended foods from each group.

SAMPLE MENU FOR YOUNG ADULTS
AGES SIXTEEN TO NINETEEN

Just as in previous stages, the calories that your child needs daily can be more or less, depending on his physical activity and growth. For example, a sedentary adolescent boy at eighteen needs 2,400 calories, and a sedentary girl at eighteen needs 1,800. On the other hand, an active adolescent boy at eighteen needs 3,200 calories, and an active adolescent girl needs 2,400. The following menu is based on a diet of 2,200 calories a day, which can be increased or lowered. You will be able to tell whether the calories your child is eating compared with those he is burning in his sports activities (or is not burning) are in balance or whether or not they are excessive and causing him to be overweight and need to be adjusted, without minimizing the importance of balanced nutrition. On the other hand, if your child eats "tons" of food and continues to be slim, then don't worry because he is probably eating the calories his body is asking him for, and needs. Something that helps parents who think their children look too *flaquitos* or skinny is to look at themselves as they were at the same age. If one of you was slender as an adolescent and battles weight now, don't pressure your child to eat more, because he could end up as overweight as you are.

	Group	Serving	Food
Breakfast	Fruit	½–1 cup	4–8 ounces cantaloupe
	Grain	1 cup	8 ounces farina
	Dairy	1 cup	8 ounces fat-free milk
Snack	Fruit	1 unit	1 medium orange
	Grain	1 slice	1 slice whole wheat bread
	Fat	1–2 teaspoons	1–2 teaspoons peanut butter or margarine (low fat)
	Various	1 teaspoon	1 teaspoon strawberry jelly
Lunch	Grain	¾–1 cup	6–8 ounces brown rice
	Protein	3 ounces	Lean beef tenderloin
	Grain	½ cup	4 ounces beans or lentils
	Vegetable	1–1½ cups	8–12 ounces vegetables: onion, *jitomate*/tomato, lettuce, green chili, cilantro
	Fat	1 tablespoon	1 tablespoon fat-free sour cream or low-fat dressing (optional)

	Group	Serving	Food
Snack	Dairy	1 cup	8 ounces fat-free milk
	Fruit	1 unit	1 medium banana
Dinner	Taco:		
	Grain	1 unit	2 corn tortillas (6 inches each)
	Protein	3 ounces	Shredded chicken without skin, baked or steamed
	Dairy	2 ounces	2–4 tablespoons shredded cheddar cheese
	Fat	1 ounce	2 tablespoons guacamole
	Vegetable	2 ounces	3–4 tablespoons tomato sauce*
		1 cup	mixed with fresh vegetables

*Tomato sauce = vegetable
Spaghetti sauce = vegetable + carbohydrate + others

At first glance the amount of foods might appear to be excessive; however, this sample menu includes the appropriate servings for all food groups, distributed throughout the day. Let your child decide how much he needs to eat. Refer to the Appendix for the daily calorie recommendations according to physical activity.

The Obese Adolescent

Obesity during adolescence can have serious repercussions on a youngster, both physically and psychologically. In the physical aspect, obese adolescents have a much higher risk of becoming obese adults, and furthermore, many of them, and especially Latinos, already have a condition known as metabolic syndrome, which indicates that their bodies are already suffering from their obesity. In the psychological sense, since this is a period in which peer acceptance is so very important, there can also be consequences in their emotional development.

BEING LEFT OUT

You have probably watched an adolescent more than once, standing before a mirror examining himself, often for a very long time. Physical appearance is very important to adolescents; how they look is one of their first priorities. You can probably still remember who were the most popular boys and girls in your class during your adolescence, and that is likely to be because of some physical characteristic and not for being *los mejores en matemáticas,* the best at math. For that reason, it is a very hard stage for obese adolescents. It is a proven fact that overweight adolescents are more often socially isolated than their companions of normal weights. Furthermore, adolescents who are the object of jokes and teasing by their companions because of their weight tend to have far less self-esteem, show more symptoms of depression, and make desperate attempts to control their weight. That is why this is the age when eating disorders begin. In the case of Latino children who have not yet adapted totally to their new culture or are having a hard time adapting, the problem of being overweight can make matters worse.

If your adolescent child is being teased for being overweight, as a parent you must recognize how important this is. It isn't something that will "go away" or that can be brushed off with a *"No les hagas caso,* don't pay attention to them," or "Just look for other friends." Your child will appreciate your help to change her eating habits and her physical activities in a healthy manner. As a professional in nutrition I recommend that you seek help aside from this book (see the Resource Guide), because in these situations sometimes parents don't have the tools necessary or the knowledge to help their child. The advice of a professional nutritionist can help a lot. It is a way to determine if your child's obesity is causing problems for him, like high cholesterol, high blood pressure, or diabetes, which are so common in Latino children at this age.

How You Can Help Your Child: Parental Attitudes

Helping an overweight adolescent generally requires a great deal of tact on the part of his parents, because on the one hand they don't take direction very easily, but on the other hand, they still need your help. In other words, they need rules and structure at the same time as they need freedom of choice. Speak to them calmly, give them information without judging them, and listen carefully. Following are some of the things you can put into practice:

- Don't make drastic changes. Strict diets tend to lead to bingeing, and this type of yo-yo dieting has the exact opposite of the desired effect on the body. Small changes, maintained over time, are the most effective.

- After beginning a new meal plan, keep a list with your child for a full week noting everything he eats during the day, along with the exact exercise he has done. Later, decide where you can begin to make healthy changes. For example, by substituting for a high-calorie snack one with fewer calories, or by watching less television and doing more exercise.

- Teach your child the benefits of a healthy diet. It is very important for her to know how to make the right decisions regarding her diet. Read this book with your child; it will help your child to understand why eating healthy is important and what effects obesity has on her body.

- Design a strategy together that will help him eat healthily if you aren't home when he comes home from school. Do the shopping together, cook and freeze proper portions for your child to use when he gets home from school.

- Talk to your child about the importance of maintaining a healthy weight, not because of how she looks on the outside, but for her health. Explain how fashion models on today's magazine covers aren't realistic. Talk to her about the importance of the values that people have on the inside.

- Praise your child for his talents and reinforce his self-esteem, especially if he is being teased at school.

- Above all, don't make negative remarks over her incapability to lose weight, her lack of willpower, or her physical appearance.

Physical Activity

If your child is like so many other adolescents, and he is "glued" to the television, Internet, or video games, encouraging him to do exercise will require a great deal of patience and creativity on your part. Physical exercise is indispensable to help him lose weight if he is already obese, or to keep him healthy, if he is not. Insufficient physical exercise is the main cause of obesity in adolescents. Encouraging your child to take part in physical activities and joining in the activity with him are the two factors, according to one study, that work the best in changing attitudes about exercise.

Outdoor family activities are an excellent way to make the whole family participate in physical exercise. Among Latinos, soccer is a favorite sport. There are many teams that play on the weekends that young people, children, and even parents can join. There are also fan clubs for many teams that organize sports activities. In the Resource Guide you will find information about contacting some of these teams. Physical activity in sports that you do with other families on weekends gives you the added benefit of establishing a relationship with other families who are also interested in physical activity.

Another way to initiate your adolescent into physical activity is to talk to her about the sports or activities she would like to practice, those within her reach. To this end, you can look into the extracurricular after-school activity programs or your local YMCA. These activities can include soccer, basketball, track, swimming, or aerobics. Learning to dance salsa is also a favorite activity for many Latino adolescents, which is something they can practice later at home. Generally, three sessions of vigorous physical activity are recommended per week. Beyond this, it is also necessary to have some sort of physical activity every day, like walking to a friend's house, helping with the housework, or simply taking the stairs instead of using the elevator. Remember that it is the small changes that we make and keep that are the most effective ones to bring more physical activity into our lives.

10

Eating Disorders: Binge Eating, Bulimia, and Anorexia

When fourteen-year-old Marta visited my practice recently, her parents were worried about "*su forma de comer,* how she ate." They wanted to talk to a nutritionist about trying to set up some healthier eating habits for her. Marta was overweight and was willing to do anything to get thinner. To achieve her objective, she decided she'd eat only once a day, at night. You can imagine what happened. By the time she got home from school she was absolutely ravenous, and she would gobble up just about all the food she could find in the house. That only made her feel guilty. To assuage her guilt, she'd eat more. She'd eat and eat and eat until she felt sick. Sometimes she tried to throw up all she'd eaten, but she wasn't always successful. Once she got swept up into the tempest of compulsive eating, she couldn't stop. So her plan to lose weight by eating only once a day actually had caused her to gain weight.

Marta's troubles are unfortunately becoming more and more common among Latina teenage girls, and even boys. Marta suffers from an eating disorder known as binge eating disorder (BED). Young Latinos also suffer from other eating disorders such as bulimia and anorexia.

Many health professionals mistakenly believe these eating disorders, especially anorexia, affect mostly white teenagers. But recent studies have shown that belief is wrong. In fact, due to certain cultural characteristics, Latina women are even more likely than whites to suffer from eating disorders.

Between 80 percent and 90 percent of the people who suffer eating disorders are teenagers, and most of them are females. The most common disorders are binge eating, bulimia, and anorexia.

Binge Eating

Up until recently, most people understood eating disorders to be either anorexia or bulimia. But over the past ten years, experts have begun to pay more attention to binge eating. More and more children, just like Marta, are binge eaters. Moreover, this eating disorder is the one that afflicts the most boys, especially Latino boys. Overweight teenagers are more likely to be binge eaters and, as we know, a high percentage of Latino teens are obese.

BINGE-EATING CHARACTERISTICS

Binge eaters frequently eat huge amounts of food all at one sitting; they feel as though they can't control themselves. These binges are often accompanied by other behaviors such as:

- Eating until they're beyond full.

- Eating huge amounts of food even though they're not hungry.

- Eating alone so others can't see how much they're eating or what foods they're eating.

- Eating much more quickly than normal.

- Feeling disgusted, guilty, or depressed after the binge.

People who suffer from bulimia can also suffer from these symptoms, but after they binge, they throw up, fast, or exercise until they're exhausted.

THE CONSEQUENCES OF BINGE EATING

Most teenage binge eaters are overweight and so the illnesses they suffer are tied to obesity: diabetes, high blood pressure, and high cholesterol levels.

People who can't control how much they eat are psychologically devastated. Most try to stop the binges, but sooner or later, they return and the cycle starts anew. Binge eaters not only feel a sense of helplessness but the extra pounds they carry also crush their self-esteem. And a low self-esteem only leads to more binges.

THE PERSONALITY OF A BINGE EATER

Binge eaters characteristically have low self-esteem. Even though on the outside they may seem very capable, both at school and at work, on the inside they usually have social problems.

Jaime was a very responsible boy, a straight-A student. However, he had almost no friends. He would hide in his room every evening and would only come out to eat. He gained a lot of weight and things got worse with time. When I cleaned his room I started noticing all kinds of empty candy wraps hiding all over. We knew it was time to ask for help.

—Carmen, forty-two years old

People who suffer from compulsive bingeing are obsessed with the guilt they feel for not being able to control their eating. Sometimes they'll avoid public gatherings to hide their binges. On some occasions, binge eaters will even skip class or work so they can eat in private.

Bulimia

Bulimia is binge eating followed by throwing up or doing something else that compensates for eating too much at once. A person suffering from bulimia can't control the desire to binge eat or the desire to throw up afterward. Bulimics may vomit, take laxatives or diuretics, or exercise to exhaustion after bingeing. They just can't help themselves.

Just like compulsive eaters, when bulimics binge, they eat far too much food in a short period of time (two hours or less). They feel as though they can't control what they're eating and afterward they feel guilt and shame for what they've done.

Although most bulimic children maintain a normal weight, they fear gaining weight. Sometimes, they'll consider themselves too fat when in fact their weight is just fine. The fact that they appear normal on the outside allows them to conceal their eating disorders longer.

THE CONSEQUENCES OF BULIMIA

Bulimia can have serious consequences because vomiting and using laxatives or diuretics can permanently damage the body. Some of the more serious consequences include:

- Tears in the esophagus and stomach, as well as distending the stomach, because so much food is eaten at once.

- Weakened tooth enamel because of the stomach acid that comes up with the vomit.

- A lack of essential minerals, such as potassium, due to excessive use of laxatives as well as throwing up.

- A higher chance of kidney stones, because of a lack of liquids; and menstrual irregularities.

THE PERSONALITY OF A BULIMIC

Just like with binge eaters, low self-esteem is a principal characteristic of bulimics.

People who suffer from bulimia may also have these problems:

- Depression.

- Mood swings.

- Impulsive behavior.

- A desire for approval.

- Little tolerance of problems.

- Difficulty relating to others.

Anorexia

Anorexic teenagers are overwhelmingly afraid of getting fat, even though they're already thin. They refuse to weigh even one pound more than what they think is the appropriate minimum for their age and height and sometimes not even that. This obsession is accompanied by a distorted perception of their own weight and their own body image; no matter what, they think they're bigger than they really are. Also, they refuse to listen to anyone who talks to them about the dangers of being too thin.

We were really desperate seeing Laura getting thinner and thinner and not being able to do anything. It didn't matter that we were constantly telling her about the consequences of her not eating. It was as if she was deaf. She would not even listen to the doctor. Finally the pediatrician gave us a referral for an eating disorders specialist.

—María Elena, thirty-nine years old

Anorexic girls will often stop menstruating. Some anorexic girls simply eat as little as possible, while others binge and then throw up or use laxatives or diuretics. Anorexics differ from bulimics in that generally they are thinner.

Curiously, at the same time anorexics deprive themselves of food, they'll enjoy cooking huge banquets for their families.

THE CONSEQUENCES OF ANOREXIA

Anorexics suffer health problems because of improper nutrition and losing too much weight. These problems include:

- Loss of menstrual cycle.

- Slow heartbeat.

- Low blood pressure.

- Appearance of body hair called lanugo because of low body temperature.

- Constipation and feeling extremely bloated after eating.

- Stunted growth.

- Anemia and a weak immune system.

Psychologically, anorexic teenager girls obsess over their weight, their appearance, and what they eat. They are also anxious, fearful, and depressed.

THE PERSONALITY OF AN ANOREXIC

Girls who are anorexic usually have an extraordinary amount of self-control and are perfectionists. At the same time, they are introverts who have a tough time establishing relationships. And as with all the other eating disorders, these girls have low self-esteem.

Unfortunately, their perfectionist personalities and excessive self-control only causes them to continue being anorexic.

People who suffer eating disorders usually have family members who suffer the same problems. A recent study showed that genetics may play a role in anorexia and bulimia. Some scientists think genes may influence up to 40 percent of these cases. However, it's likely that social factors, such as the pressure to look good or to follow strict diets at young ages, activate these genes.

Factors Contributing to Eating Disorders Among Young Latinas

Most of us have seen family photo albums with those tattered black-and-white pictures showing an *abuelita o bisabuela,* grandmother or great-grandmother, dressed in stern clothing—you know, those dark-colored high-necked dresses. These photos usually show serious women who are a little on the heavy side surrounded by their families, or even holding babies in their arms. These pictures give us a good idea about what the ideal woman was: a mother who sacrificed everything for her family.

But in the 1920s, things began to change, especially for women in the United States. Thin was in. Having a svelte body meant being in favor of all the new rights and privileges women were assuming at that time: the right to vote and work and be independent. This was a move away from the Victorian image of a woman. During the 1960s, thinness was taken to the extreme, and the ideal woman became nearly skeletal. This desire to be thin remains with us today. Today's image of the beautiful woman is presented constantly in the movies, magazines, and music videos, and there's no doubt the ideal woman is thin. Many of these women are even thinner than the average woman, or their Ideal Body Weight.

For a long time, this idea of thin being beautiful didn't really affect young Latina girls because for us Latinas, beauty was more about being a good mother and wife, who was curvier than the superthin models seen in the United States and Europe. However, some studies have shown that eating disorders affect Latina girls more than others, especially overweight Latinas. Surveys say Latina girls are more likely to be binge eaters and depressed.

Low Self-Esteem and Poor Body Image

Most people who suffer eating disorders have previously developed low self-esteem and poor body image. Puberty brings with it wider hips and other natural changes that result in a larger body. So when these Latina girls get to their teenage years, they're terribly unhappy with their bodies and feel even worse about themselves.

Young women between the ages of thirteen and eighteen make up 90 percent of all the cases of eating disorders. A girl who develops eating disorders often just can't accept these natural changes that are turning her into a woman, and in the case of many Latina girls, a full-figured woman. The physical features of most Latina women aren't the same as the ones of the ideal Anglo beauties the media constantly shows us. In addition, many Latina girls are obese and studies have shown overweight young people are more likely to develop eating disorders, especially binge eating.

Young People Torn Between Latino and Anglo Cultures

Many young Latina girls in the United States often find themselves torn between two contradictory cultures because at this age they probably haven't discovered who they are. So they're more susceptible to falling into the trap of eating disorders. A common scenario is the young girl living in a home where her parents are strict Latinos, who only speak Spanish and adhere to their native traditions. Meanwhile, the daughter would like nothing better than to be a part of her English-speaking group of friends, speaking only English, dressing in the most hip clothes, and wearing makeup advertised in popular American magazines.

> *It was as if Isabel had forgotten completely that she was Latina. She didn't even want to be called Isabel anymore! Now she was Elizabeth and would only speak English, even at home. It made me sad, this rejection of who we are.*
>
> *—Sylvia, forty years old*

Young girls who feel they have to hide part of their own culture in order to be accepted by their friends find themselves conflicted; they feel bad about themselves and begin to feel anxious. This sad circumstance is really common among girls who've just arrived in the United States and left behind grandparents or other loved ones in their home country. This stress is a big factor in developing eating disorders.

In general, children are less likely to suffer eating disorders if:

- They feel proud and have a connection with their own community.

- Their idea of what's beautiful includes full-figured bodies.

- Their self-esteem is based more on spiritual values than in material possessions, or physical appearance.

DOES MY CHILD HAVE AN EATING DISORDER?

Many Latino families have a difficult time accepting the fact that their daughter or son has an uncontrollable eating disorder. Mental illnesses and behavioral problems elicit little sympathy among Latinos. Generally, we Latinos think overcoming eating problems is a matter of self-control and *voluntad,* will. Other times, it's the parents who refuse to believe their daughter could have an eating disorder because they don't want to face up to the shame and pain of the problem.

Eating disorders aren't easy to overcome. If it were only a question of wanting to, there would be far fewer young girls who suffer from them. For example, binge eating is a compulsion—the person who suffers really can't help it; she doesn't have any control over how much she eats, no matter how much she wants to stop. The same happens with bulimia and anorexia; children who suffer from these diseases really can't stop vomiting or really can't eat more, even though they know it's affecting their physical and mental health.

The first step in helping your daughter is knowing for sure she's got an eating disorder. If you think she may be ill, don't accept her saying, "Oh, *todo está bien,* everything's okay," or "*Ya me va a pasar,* I'll get over it." Nor should you listen to other family members who say, "It comes with being a teenager." Some of the behaviors that may tell you your daughter has an eating disorder include:

- Obsessively counting calories or fat grams.

- Being on a continuous diet.

- Refusing to sit at the table with the family during dinner.

- Going to the bathroom right after eating.

- Missing menstrual periods.

- Losing a lot of weight in a short period of time.

- Exercising excessively or undertaking other activities to constantly burn calories.

- Taking laxatives or diuretics.

- Hiding their actual weight under "big clothes."

There's also a chance you may find entire boxes of food missing from the refrigerator or pantry. If the gallon of ice cream or box of cereal or tin of cookies you bought for the entire family disappears, ask who ate it and watch for your daughter's reaction. She may be suffering from an eating disorder.

THE FAMILY'S REACTION TO EATING DISORDERS

The way you and your family react to your daughter's eating disorder is critical. Generally, when parents figure out what's going on, a war breaks out over the behavior of the ill person. If the daughter suffers from anorexia, families will start an all-out campaign to make sure she eats. If the disorder is binge eating, the family will try to keep food from her.

As well-meaning as these attitudes are, they're useless, if not counterproductive. They rarely cure the disorder, and even worse, they create more anxiety for the entire family. There are other things the family can do to help:

- Talk to your daughter about her worries. Listen but don't judge.

- Think about how your family deals with and reacts to thinness. Does your family diet frequently? Your daughter may believe that if she's not thin she's not worthy of being loved.

- Talk about physical and emotional health, not about weight and body size.

- Get help. The Resource Guide shows you where to find information about and treatment for eating disorders. Remember, only a doctor or a mental health professional can diagnose eating disorders, and the sooner they're treated, the better the chances of success.

If anything, don't blame the person who suffers an eating disorder. Look for professional help and try to relate food to physical health and not to physical appearance.

11

Illnesses: Consequences of Obesity

How to Manage Type 2 Diabetes, High Cholesterol, and High Blood Pressure in Children

Within traditional Latino culture, it's hard to accept that a child could actually be sick just from being overweight. Carrying a few extra pounds during childhood is actually seen as a sign of strength or *ser fuerte*. One recent study showed that even though overweight children want to lose the extra pounds so their friends will be more accepting of them, these same children also consider themselves healthier and stronger than thinner children. While many parents do know that obesity causes certain illnesses, they wrongly believe these problems only happen to adults.

Obese children can indeed suffer many health problems just because they're overweight. For the longest time, doctors thought type 2 diabetes was a disease that only affected adults older than forty, but now it's showing up among obese children, especially Latino children. Years ago it was rare for pediatricians to come across children with type 2 diabetes. Today, it's rare to find an obese Latino child who *doesn't* suffer from type 2 diabetes, high blood pressure, or high cholesterol. In fact, 90 percent of all children who have some difficulty producing insulin or who have high levels of fats in their blood are overweight.

These illnesses, especially diabetes, can be devastating to a child's life. Having fun—going to a birthday party, playing soccer, or spending the night with a friend—now suddenly has to be carefully planned out. Children with diabetes have to look forward every day to pricking a finger to draw blood to test sugar levels and adjusting what they eat depending on the test results. As if that weren't complicated enough, this disease makes them different from their friends, which can cause emotional and behavioral problems, especially among teenagers.

The good news is that these illnesses can be controlled by following a healthy diet and exercise, though of course under proper medical supervision.

Your child may already be obese, but it's likely you still don't know if the extra pounds have caused any health problems. In this chapter, you'll find a guide to help you identify the most common illnesses caused by obesity: type 2 diabetes, high cholesterol, and high blood pressure. However, always remember, only a doctor has the right tools to determine whether your child is indeed sick. The Resource Guide has information on where to get help.

Type 2 Diabetes

Obese Latino children suffer from type 2 diabetes more than any other chronic illness. Being overweight is the principle reason for this situation, but in the case of Latino children, a lack of exercise and a genetic predisposition toward diabetes makes them even more vulnerable. That is, Latino children have genes that make them more likely to be diabetic, and being overweight and not exercising only makes the likelihood even higher. That's why if you or your spouse is diabetic or you've got close relatives who are, and your child is overweight, you should talk to a doctor to find out if your child has diabetes. This is important because for every child who has already developed type 2 diabetes, there are several others who have what's called metabolic syndrome (a combination of obesity, insulin resistance, high triglycerides, and high blood pressure), a disease that especially afflicts Latino children. A child with metabolic syndrome is much more likely to develop type 2 diabetes.

What Is Type 2 Diabetes?

Diabetes is an illness that prevents people from properly metabolizing the food they eat.

Human beings eat so that the cells in our bodies can have the nourishment they need to carry out different functions. The digestive process converts the food we eat into a sugar called glucose. This sugar is the fuel our cells burn as they do their jobs. When cells are well nourished, that means we've got enough energy to live and breathe and do the things we want to do.

In order for cells to burn glucose, they need insulin, which is produced by the pancreas. Think of insulin as the key that unlocks the cap to the cell's fuel tank. If there's not enough insulin, the cap won't come off and the glucose can't get into the fuel tank.

People with diabetes don't produce enough insulin, or their bodies can't use it properly. Glucose, or sugar, can't get into the cells, and so it stays in the bloodstream.

There are various types of diabetes:

Type 1 diabetes: People with this type of diabetes produce very little insulin or none at all. For reasons scientists still can't figure out, the immune system destroys the cells that produce insulin inside the pancreas. Symptoms are severe and patients need daily insulin injections just to survive. This type of diabetes usually appears before the age of twenty.

Type 2 diabetes: Most diabetics have this form of the disease. It's also the most common among Latinos. Type 2 diabetics do produce insulin, but their bodies can't use it properly or the pancreas can't produce enough insulin.

Gestational diabetes: This type of diabetes occurs only during pregnancy. The hormones in the placenta block insulin and stop glucose from entering cells.

There are other types of diabetes caused by pancreas disorders or by certain medicines.

Certain conditions can appear before diabetes actually begins:

Insulin resistance: Insulin no longer has any effect on cells (it doesn't unlock the fuel cap to allow in glucose) so the pancreas begins to make more and more insulin, trying to reduce the glucose levels in the bloodstream. This vicious circle continues until the pancreas fails because it's tried too hard to produce insulin. Then when it really can't produce any more, diabetes kicks in. Obese Latino children are more likely than others to develop insulin resistance.

Glucose intolerance: This is related to insulin resistance. Because the insulin isn't working (it isn't unlocking the fuel caps), it remains in the bloodstream in high levels, although not as high as it gets in the case of diabetes. According to one study, 28 percent of overweight Latino children also have glucose intolerance, even though they haven't developed diabetes yet.

THE CONSEQUENCES OF TYPE 2 DIABETES
IN CHILDREN

High levels of sugar or insulin in the blood can damage veins and nerves in vital organs, such as the kidneys, heart, and eyes.

The more time a person goes without receiving treatment for diabetes, the greater the chances are for developing these complications. For example, adults who develop diabetes may go as long as ten to fourteen years without feeling the effects. In other words, if a person gets diabetes at forty-five years of age, without proper treatment their organs will start to be damaged by the age of fifty-five or sixty. But if the diabetes begins at age ten or fifteen and goes untreated, then the damage to the organs will begin to appear at age twenty to twenty-five, just when a young person is generally beginning a first job or having children.

Doctors are now treating teenagers who are suffering serious problems from diabetes. These problems are generally irreversible.

The first complications that appear in children who get diabetes include:

- High cholesterol.

- High blood pressure.

- Irregular menstrual periods or polycystic ovarian syndrome.

- Acantosis nigricans, or dark patches around the neck and armpits.

SIGNS THAT YOUR CHILD MAY HAVE TYPE 2 DIABETES

A case of diabetes can only be confirmed by doing a blood test after the patient drinks a special cocktail made of glucose. However, certain symptoms may indicate that your child has diabetes. For example, if your child is obese, if you or your spouse is diabetic or if you have diabetic relatives, or if dark patches of skin suddenly appear on your child's neck or armpits, there might be a strong possibility that your child has diabetes. Other physical characteristics that can indicate a case of type 2 diabetes include early sexual development, excessive hair on females, irregular menstruation, being unusually tall, and having strong body odor.

There are other signs to look out for that may indicate that your child has diabetes:

- Does your child urinate frequently, getting up several times during the night?

- In school, have your child's teachers noticed an unusual number of requests to get a drink of water because of persistent thirst?

- Is your child worn out after school? Are *siestas* a necessity?

- Does your child have frequent urinary tract infections, or in the case of a daughter, does she have many vaginal infections (does she feel burning when urinating or do her panties have a strong odor and is there excessive vaginal discharge)?

- Do simple cuts or bruises on the skin take a long time to heal?

- Does your child feel dizzy at times?

- Does your child have blurred vision?

High cholesterol and high blood pressure are other signs of diabetes. Normal blood glucose levels are between 80 and 120 mg/dl before meals and not more than 140 mg/dl after meals. However, these values vary from child to child. That's why it's so important to consult a doctor to figure out exactly which levels are appropriate for your child.

How to Manage Type 2 Diabetes
in Children and Adolescents

It's virtually impossible to get a child or teenager to understand just how serious the consequences are of having type 2 diabetes. So when a child does suffer this illness, it's important to try to include in the treatment many of the people who come in contact with the child: brothers, sisters, aunts, uncles, teachers, school nurses, coaches, and counselors. Controlling diabetes isn't just the child's responsibility. Education is one of the best tools to battle diabetes, not only for the child but also for parents.

Scientists are right now working on possible cures for diabetes, including genetic therapies, transplanting the cells that produce insulin in the pancreas, and even artificial pancreases. However, the sad reality is that today there is no cure for this illness and the only way to deal with it is to try to control it day by day.

To control diabetes, every day a child must:

- *Follow a diet recommended by a doctor, nutritionist or diabetes educator*: The plan will help to ensure sugar levels in the blood remain constant. Children and the rest of the family must be able to recognize different types of food and how they affect blood sugar levels. For example, complex carbohydrates such as rice, tortillas, pasta, or bread will change blood sugar levels more than other types of foods. The number and size of the portions of these foods, even though they're considered healthy, can also alter blood sugar levels. Sugar levels are also controlled by monitoring how often the child eats and how much time passes between meals. A good diet for the diabetic child includes different foods from different levels of the Latino food pyramid, in the appropriate portions, as well as a sufficient amount of fiber, low fat and cholesterol, low sodium (i.e., salt), and hardly any sweets. Avoiding sodas, sweets, *postres,* and cereals high in sugar is essential.

- *Exercise regularly*: Children and teenagers who have diabetes need to exercise on a regular basis to help control their blood sugar levels. However, be careful to ensure blood sugar levels aren't too low before the exercise begins, because that can lead to other problems. Your doctor will tell you what type of exercise, when, how often, and for how long, is best for your child.

- *Monitor glucose levels every day*: A glucose monitor reads the amount of glucose in the blood. A droplet of blood is extracted by pricking the tip of your child's finger. This is uncomfortable for children, but there are various types of blood extractors with really fine lancets that make the pricks bearable. Staying on top of blood glucose levels is key to controlling diabetes, because the goal here is to avoid the really high levels of sugar in the blood that can damage organs and cause other complications. To have your child monitor his blood sugar levels at school, you'll need a note from the doctor and a parental permission form.

- *Take prescribed medicines at the right time and in the right amount*: If a good diet and exercise alone aren't enough to control your child's diabetes, you may need to include drugs in the treatment. If your child must take these medicines during the school day, talk to the teachers and school nurses to make sure everyone's helping to do what's best for your child.

In addition to a balanced diet, your doctor may recommend that your child lose weight. When people lose weight, their cells become much more sensitive to the effects of insulin. In other words, after losing weight, the insulin secreted by the pancreas may be enough on its own to reduce blood sugar levels.

> *I felt different after following my meal program. Before I was always tired and in a bad mood. It takes some work to pay attention at all the new rules I have for my eating but I'd rather feel like I feel now than before, even if I was eating more of the stuff I like.*
>
> *—Diego, sixteen years old*

If your child is still in the growing stages, any diet to lose weight must be recommended and supervised by a pediatrician or nutritionist. A diet whose purpose is to control diabetes should be personalized for each child. It's important to get help from a doctor or nutritionist to make sure your child is following a plan that can lead to success. In the Resource Guide you will find help.

If your child eats the lunch offered at the school cafeteria, it may be difficult to say no to a hamburger or slice of pizza, especially if there are no healthy, tasty alternatives such as vegetables and fresh salads.

Think about it: If the only options were an apple, a pear, or a banana, you can bet a child would always choose something healthy. But the reality is that the choices are more likely to be doughnuts, potato chips, or soda, none of which offers much nutritional value. Only parents can pressure schools to offer children healthy food choices.

Don't be afraid to exercise your rights. There are federal and state laws that protect disabled children, including children with diabetes. Diabetic children have access to programs, at both public and private schools. Also, you've got the right to demand that the school make changes so your child is safe and healthy at school. Diabetic children have the same right to an education as other children. Still, your child will best learn how to control diabetes at home.

Finally, don't forget that managing diabetes can be stressful, for the parents and the child. Be alert for signs of depression and eating disorders.

High Cholesterol

Obesity and diabetes both result in high levels of cholesterol in the blood. If a blood test has shown that your child has high cholesterol, it's likely your pediatrician will check for diabetes, and vice versa; if your child has diabetes, the doctor will check cholesterol levels.

What Is High Cholesterol?

Cholesterol is a fatty substance that looks like wax. Our bodies need it for all kinds of important functions, such as creating new cells. The so-called bad cholesterol, or LDL, accumulates on the inside of blood vessels and can cause serious damage to the brain, heart, and kidneys.

Cholesterol flows through the bloodstream, but it doesn't dissolve in blood. So it moves around by attaching itself to particles called lipoproteins. There are several types of lipoproteins, but the ones you've most likely heard about are:

Bad cholesterol, or LDL (low-density lipoproteins). This type of lipoprotein carries cholesterol from the liver to various body tissues. The
problem is, along the way cholesterol is left behind, deposited on the
walls of blood vessels. If enough gets stuck to the inside of the vessel
walls, the entire vessel can become blocked. So-called bad cholesterol
is produced in the liver and can be introduced in the body through the
foods we eat (fatty meats, cheeses, *embutidos*, etc.). Cholesterol from
food is known as dietery cholesterol.

Good cholesterol, or HDL (high-density lipoproteins). This type of
lipoprotein is known as the good cholesterol because it helps to eliminate excess bad cholesterol from the interior walls of arteries and
veins. This lipoprotein carries cholesterol from various parts of the
body back to the liver, where it's discarded as waste. That's why some
people call HDL the "vacuum cleaner for the bad cholesterol." Exercise and a diet high in fiber and low in fat and dietary cholesterol increases the amount of HDL in your body.

CONSEQUENCES OF HIGH CHOLESTEROL

Atherosclerosis is an illness that occurs when the cholesterol and fats
that flow through the bloodstream accumulate in the form of plaque
inside blood vessels. This plaque buildup reduces the amount of oxygen these vessels can send to body tissues. Sometimes a chunk of
plaque will break loose and a blood clot is created than can completely
block a vein or artery. When this happens, no blood flows through the
vessel at all, and whatever tissues are on the other side of the blockage
don't get any oxygen at all. This is dangerously harmful for that part of
the body. If this affected body part is the heart or brain, the damage
can be fatal. In fact, in most Western countries, this is the number one
cause of death, much more common than other diseases.

Today we know atherosclerosis begins in infancy and slowly gets worse
as we become adults. Cholesterol levels during infancy are an important
factor in determining the likelihood that an adult will have this disease.

Signs Your Child Could Have High Cholesterol

High cholesterol is a silent disease. There are no symptoms until the levels are dangerously high. However, there are certain signs you can look for: If your children have diabetes, they probably have high cholesterol too. Also, don't forget cholesterol levels are not only affected by the food we eat but also by the child's weight and by heredity. Your family has a history of high cholesterol if you or your spouse, a grandparent or aunt or uncle has had one of the following before the age of fifty-five: a heart attack, angina, atherosclerosis, sudden death from heart disease, or cholesterol levels above 240 mg/dL.

On the other hand, certain illnesses such as hyperthyroidism or kidney or liver disease can cause high cholesterol levels.

For children and teenagers ages two to nineteen, the following are acceptable levels of cholesterol:

Level	Total cholesterol (mg / dl)	LDL cholesterol (mg / dl)
Acceptable	Less than 170	Less than 110
Limit	170–199	110–129
High	200 or more	130 or more

Also, the levels of HDL (the good cholesterol) should be at least 35 mg/dL or higher, and the levels of triglycerides (another type of fat that circulates through the bloodstream and can cause heart disease) should be 150 mg/dL or less.

How to Manage High Cholesterol in Children and Teenagers

Nutritionists have proven that if children and teenagers follow a balanced diet with the appropriate number of calories, they can reduce their levels of LDL cholesterol without stunting their growth or development.

In addition to controlling their weight, these children should also exercise between thirty and sixty minutes a day, or nearly every day. Aerobic exercise is any type of activity that causes an increase in both respiration and heart rate: jumping, running, cycling, walking, or swimming.

Diets designed to control cholesterol for children should have no more than 30 percent of the calories coming from fats, and cholesterol intake should not be higher than 300 mg per day, according to government health agencies.

More than anything, the child should avoid trans fats and saturated fats. Food labels will tell you the exact amount of both fats.

Some tips to reduce fats in your child's diet include:

- Use low-fat meats for cooking as well as in sandwiches.

- Exchange whole milk for skim milk. This simple change can really cut down on fat intake.

- Always read food labels and understand just how much trans fats, saturated fats, and cholesterol are in the food you're eating.

- Use cooking methods that are low in fat, such as broiling, boiling, grilling, steaming, etc.

All these recommendations about the appropriate amounts of cholesterol and fats in your child's diet are included the Latino food pyramid in Chapter Four and in the sample menus in the chapters dealing with age-appropriate foods.

Just as with diabetes, controlling cholesterol is work for the whole family. Children and teenagers need help to have balanced nutrition, choose the right foods, and exercise the right amount. Smoking is definitely a no-no, because it only makes atherosclerosis and other diseases worse.

If your doctor determines that diet and exercise are not enough to control cholesterol, you may need to include medications in the treatment. Some drugs for children older than ten can help to lower cholesterol, but they need to be closely monitored by a physician.

High Blood Pressure or Hypertension

You may think high blood pressure is a problem only adults have to deal with, but unfortunately this is not true. The explosion of obesity among children has brought with it an increase in high blood pressure, or hypertension, among children. In fact, high blood pressure is nine times more common among obese children than among children of normal weight. A lack of exercise, high sodium (i.e., salt) intake, and diabetes are among the causes of high blood pressure.

WHAT IS HIGH BLOOD PRESSURE?

Blood pressure is the pressure that blood exerts on the interior walls of vessels as it's pumped through by the heart. A normal blood pressure reading is about 120/80 mm of Hg (the number of millimeters that the mercury rises on the gauge in a blood-pressure test). These numbers measure the pressure. The heart is a hollow muscle that pushes out blood as it contracts. The contraction phase of the heartbeat is called systole, and that causes the pressure to go up. The first number of the test reading is higher and records blood pressure at its highest point. This is called maximum, or systolic, pressure.

The second number measures the pressure at the moment the heart relaxes and isn't pumping (diastole). This measurement is known as minimum, or diastolic, pressure. This cycle of contraction and relaxation occurs in less than a second; it's what happens as you feel your heart beat.

Arterial pressure depends on the amount of blood the heart is pumping through the vessels and the ability of the arteries and veins to stretch to accommodate the blood flow. Think of how water flows through the garden hose. The more water you force through the hose and the less flexible the hose is, the more pressure there is. The higher the blood pressure, the harder the heart has to work to move blood through the body. Fatty tissue requires a lot of blood, so the more overweight a person is, the more blood there is and the harder the body has to work to pump it.

CONSEQUENCES OF HIGH BLOOD PRESSURE OR HYPERTENSION

High blood pressure means the heart and the veins and arteries have to work harder, constantly. That's why this disease must be treated right away, before permanent damage is done to the heart and the blood vessels. If not, the problems could include kidney and brain hemorrhages.

The constant extra effort the heart has to exert can make it larger, especially the left ventricle—a chamber of the heart. Latino children are more likely to suffer from this problem. And an enlarged left ventricle makes heart attacks more likely in the future.

All these risks only emphasize why it's so important to have your doctor determine if your child has high blood pressure and whether the heart has suffered any damage. Doctors determine heart size through echocardiograms, which is like a sonogram but for the heart.

High blood pressure in children is related to insulin resistance, which as we know disproportionately affects Latino children. Several studies have shown high blood pressure during infancy is a sure predictor of high blood pressure in adulthood, and all the accompanying damage to the heart and other vital organs. Several factors that cause high blood pressure in adults originate during infancy. Some of them include:

- Obesity during infancy.

- High sodium intake during infancy.

- Not breastfeeding.

■ Mother's high blood pressure during pregnancy.

■ Mother's smoking during pregnancy.

Signs That Your Child Could Have High Blood Pressure

This condition doesn't cause discomfort right away, making it difficult to detect. In fact, the only way to measure it is with a gauge called a sphygmomanometer, that gadget the doctor wraps around your arm and then squeezes the rubber ball to increase the pressure.

There are some symptoms that can indicate a problem with high blood pressure:

■ Headaches

■ Vision problems

■ Dizziness

■ Fatigue

Generally, a pediatrician will discover that a child has high blood pressure during an office visit. That's because checking blood pressure is part of most routine visits. You should have your child's blood pressure checked at least once a year, especially if your child is overweight or has diabetes.

If your doctor discovers that your child has high blood pressure, the next step will probably be further tests to make sure no other problems exist besides obesity. There may be a problem with the heart, the kidneys, or the endocrine system.

The pediatrician will probably take your child's blood pressure several times. Because children are nervous at the beginning of the visit, their blood pressure readings tend to be higher soon after arriving at the office. Blood pressure can also vary according to age, sex, and height. Below you'll find a reference chart to find which readings are normal for your child's age.

The first figure in each column refers to systolic pressure, and the second, to diastolic pressure (< means *less than*; < = means *less than or equal to*; > means *more than*; >= means *more than or equal to*).

	Boys		Girls	
Age	*Normal*	*High*	*Normal*	*High*
1	< 103/54	>= 106/58	< 103/56	>= 107/60
2 to 3	< 109/63	>= 113/67	< 106/65	>= 110/69
4 to 5	< 112/70	>= 116/74	< 109/70	>= 113/74
6 to 7	< 115/74	>= 119/78	< 113/73	>= 116/77
8 to 10	< 119/78	>= 123/82	< 118/76	>= 122/80
11 to 12	< 123/79	>= 127/83	< 122/78	>= 133/90
13 to 14	< 128/80	>= 132/84	< 125/80	>= 136/92
15 to 17	< 136/84	>= 140/89	< 128/82	>= 132/86

After age eighteen, the values are the same for teenagers and adults:

Normal: <= 120/80
High: >= 140/90

Sometimes, the readings will fall between normal and high. This is called prehypertension, or in other words, the first step on the way to having high blood pressure.

How to Manage High Blood Pressure in Children and Teenagers

One of the first steps you should take to try to reduce high blood pressure in your children is to cut back on sodium in their diet. That includes the salt you use to cook, to season dishes at the table, soy sauce and bottle sauces, processed cheeses, smoked meats, and bouillon cubes, as well as the sodium that comes in prepared foods. Look for the word *sodium* on the nutrition labels. That's what we commonly refer to as salt. However, sodium is not only found in salt but in many other food condiments. If the hypertension isn't too bad, this simple strategy may control it.

In addition to watching how much salt you add to foods, you should carefully watch for the sodium contained in canned and prepackaged foods. The caffeine that sodas contain can also increase blood pressure, and Latino children drink more soda than any other group of children in the country.

Weight loss is another strategy to reduce blood pressure. When an obese child loses the extra weight, blood pressure generally returns to normal. That's why eating a balanced diet and regular exercise are the first recommendations your doctor will make.

If these strategies don't work, and your child's blood pressure stays high, there are certain medications your doctor can prescribe. Treating high blood pressure in children is important to prevent the long-term damage it does to organs.

And just because your child's blood pressure does come down after reducing salt or sodium intake, eating a balanced diet, getting regular exercise, and/or taking some medications, that doesn't mean you should quit taking all the precautions. High blood pressure is something that can come back as soon as the bad habits return.

All the illnesses described in this chapter can be difficult to deal with, not only for the children and teenagers who suffer from them but also for their families. The most important thing is to remember that many of these problems can be controlled or eliminated with the right treatment. In the end, the changes you should make will help not only your child but the entire family lead a healthier life.

12

María, Raúl, and Theresa: Three Stories of Success

M any Latino families with overweight children come to my office every year. Not all of these families have the same challenges. Sometimes they have a diabetic child; other times the child has not developed serious health problems, but they have a high risk to have them soon. But in all cases, families and children face the challenge to make changes in their daily routines and lead a healthier life.

Very often, it is not just the child who has to change his eating behaviors and style of life: The whole family has to make the change, and sometimes this is not easy. However, with the proper information, support, and monitoring, the large majority of families I assist achieve their goals.

In this chapter I want to share with you three cases very representative of the problems that affect overweight Latino children today:

María, an overweight seven-year-old girl; Raúl, a fourteen-year-old diabetic boy, and Theresa, a twelve-year-old preadolescent with eating disorders.

María: Inadequate Diet and Too Much Soda

María came to my office with her parents because their pediatrician told them to consult with a nutritionist. María weighed too much for her age and height. The pediatrician feared the excess weight would interfere with the correct development of her leg bones and cause orthopedic problems in the future. In addition, María had some signs of prediabetes. If she didn't change her habits she could end up having full-blown diabetes.

María's parents, just like many other Latino parents, were not very convinced that María's extra weight was a serious problem. Although they admitted María was a little bit *gordita*, chubby, they didn't think it was something to worry about. They believed María would lose the weight when she grew up. In fact, according to our culture, María's weight had a "healthy" aspect. They told me María's maternal grandmother, a woman who had raised seven children successfully, didn't think María had any problem—just the opposite: "She looked like a very healthy and strong girl."

During several visits we talked about the traditional wisdom of our culture that thinks a *gordito* child is a healthy one, and how things have changed. They agreed that today looking *gordito* is not necessarily an indication of good health. We saw that María's medical evaluations showed that her development could be affected by her excess weight, and we talked about her signs of prediabetes. María's paternal grandmother was diabetic and María's father knew well the consequences of the disease. His mother had gone blind and several of her toes had had to be amputated because her blood sugar levels were not properly controlled.

Through our interviews María's parents also understood that they didn't have to put María on a diet so she would lose weight, nor did they have to forbid her to eat the things she liked. María's mother liked to cook, and although she didn't have a lot of time on her hands, she often prepared her family's favorite *platillos*, dishes.

For a week María and her parents wrote down their activities and meals so we could later analyze the changes we would progressively introduce to improve María's diet and physical activity, as well as all the family.

A typical sample menu for María was:

Breakfast	Cereal high in added sugars and low in fiber, with whole milk
Lunch	Wheat flour quesadilla with beef, canned sugared fruit, and packaged flavored drinks
Snack	Chocolate cookies with cream filling and a regular soda
Dinner	Macaroni and cheese, tamales, and a regular soda; fresh vegetables (rarely)
Snack	Chocolate ice cream with cookies

We made several changes in María's menu that greatly reduced the number of calories. She was able to adapt easily to these changes:

Breakfast	Cereal with low to moderate added sugar and with fiber; skim milk
Lunch	Corn flour quesadilla with lean meat; fresh fruit and sugar-free soda (with the goal of choosing healthier beverages later)
Snack	Low-sodium crackers with cheese and 100 percent juice or a fresh fruit and water

Dinner	Spaghetti with tomato sauce and sprinkled with cheese and/or low-fat enchiladas, mixed salad, and a glass of skim milk
Snack	Fat-free frozen yogurt

These changes reduced the number of calories and increased the nutrients in María's diet. Now we had to slowly introduce vegetables, keep and/or increase the low-fat dairy products, and substitute the sodas with natural beverages such as juices with no added sugar or *aguas frescas*, fruit-flavored water. As the weeks went by, and thanks to a good dose of patience, perseverance, and imagination on the part of María's parents, she started accepting vegetables in her diet, cooked and fresh, up to the recommended servings for her age. María even told me that she was proud of herself for liking vegetables.

DAILY SERVINGS FOR
CHILDREN AGES SIX TO EIGHT

Food groups	Amount
Grains, legumes	2½–3 cups
Vegetables	2 cups or more
Fruit	2–2½ cups/units
Low-fat milk	3 cups
Lean protein	4–6 ounces
Healthy fats	1½–2 tablespoons

However, there was an area that was more difficult to change: drinking soda. María was used to drinking soda and although she was tolerating the sugarless kind, every day she would drink between four and five servings. Forcing María, or any child her age, not to drink soda from the refrigerator at home does not work. Furthermore, it can produce unnecessary fights. María's parents adopted several rules that ended up producing results:

- They stopped buying soda. In the refrigerator María could only find *aguas frescas*, natural juices, and water.

- They didn't give María money to buy soda at school. Instead they gave her other options, like bringing small bottles of water or packaged four-ounce juices (100 percent) from home.

- They allowed María to have sodas occasionally when they went out for dinner or on special occasions.

Although it was not easy at the beginning, María and her family slowly accepted the changes in their diet. At the same time they increased their physical activity. After dinner they would go out with María for a walk, or they would play for a while in the park outside. On the weekends they tried to plan more physical activities for everybody.

After a few months, the change in María's weight was visible; the prediabetes was under control and in general the family had a much healthier life that showed in their level of health and energy.

Raúl: Controlling Diabetes

Raúl's mother suspected something was wrong with her son. The last few months he had complained of always being tired, drank soda constantly, and got up to urinate several times every night. Raúl was fourteen years old and overweight. Although his parents tried to control his diet, their attempts were not very successful. He ate all kinds of snacks between meals and his mother felt bad about stopping him. His parents were not very concerned about his weight. They thought of him as a "strong" boy.

During a routine medical checkup, Raúl's mother told the pediatrician the symptoms she observed in her son. After a few tests it was confirmed that Raúl had developed type 2 diabetes. Raúl's mother had had gestational diabetes during pregnancy, but she couldn't imagine that an adolescent would be able to have the disease.

When they came to see me they thought the diabetes would go away with treatment. They were upset when they learned that was not the case; it is possible to control diabetes but the disease will not "go away." However they were relieved to know that they had detected the illness very early, and with the proper diet and the right lifestyle, Raúl would be able to avoid serious consequences for his health in the future, and also lead a healthier life.

The plan to treat Raúl's diabetes had three basic points:

- Follow a meal plan in order to maintain stable blood sugar levels

- Exercise daily or regularly

- Measure blood sugar levels, daily if possible

Regarding Raúl's diet, he was used to eating vegetables and fruits during his meals. His problem was that he was hungry all the time and was constantly eating sugary and high-calorie snacks. We planned a menu with the right calories for Raúl and with three meals and three healthy snacks in between to maintain his blood sugar levels. The menu and the mealtimes prevented his blood sugar from spiking up or down; the more organized the menu and mealtimes, the more controlled are blood sugar levels. After a few weeks Raúl's blood sugar levels were stabilized, the hunger had disappeared, and his diet was much healthier.

However, the other two parts of the treatment were more difficult to follow. Raúl was a TV and video game addict and it was almost impossible to make him exercise. The first thing his parents did was to register him in an after-school sports program offered in his district. Raúl was not very happy with the idea, but he was feeling much better now that his blood sugar levels were controlled, and he was eventually able to be part of the activities. Some afternoons they played soccer and others they played basketball. Raúl, like his father, loved soccer. Now in addition to watching soccer games on TV he was able to practice the sport himself. Also, his father found a local team where fathers and sons played soccer on weekends and where they could share their passion with other people.

The part that was giving Raúl more trouble, and also troubling his parents, was the daily finger pricking to measure his blood sugar. Raúl had always been scared about pricking and needles and they had a daily battle in order to measure his blood sugar level. After several weeks of fighting I recommended that they try other easier methods to measure the blood sugar, if their pediatrician approved. There are some blood sugar monitors that obtain the blood droplet from the forearm, which is less painful than getting it from the fingertips. Raúl tried the monitor and taking his blood measurements become much easier.

Today Raúl's diabetes is under control, his weight is returning to normal, and he feels much better. Raúl's disease brought some healthy changes for his family too. Thanks to the Saturday soccer games his father has also lost weight, he feels healthier, and he now has a closer relationship with his son.

Theresa: The Beginning of Eating Disorders

Twelve-year-old Theresa and her parents were well aware of her weight problem when they came to see me. Theresa was very overweight for her height and age, and that was affecting her self-esteem and performance at school. Some days Theresa was refusing to go to school because her classmates teased her.

The relationship with her parents was also tense. Theresa went from strict dieting to bingeing. Her mother had found her several times vomiting in the bathroom after she'd just eaten. Theresa's parents blamed her for her inability to control her appetite, but aside from the blaming, they really didn't know how to help her. They were very worried about how avoiding class because of her weight could affect her studies, her future, and her health.

Theresa's parents were both obese. There were always sweets and sodas in the refrigerator. Her favorite entertainment was to watch TV or to have dinner in a restaurant. The most difficult part in Theresa's case was to convince the family that Theresa's "problem" was not just *her* problem. The whole family had to participate in the solution, and that meant changing their way of eating and starting to exercise. They also had to accept that Theresa was starting to develop an eating disorder known as bulimia, which if not treated could have serious physiological and psychological consequences in the future.

It was not easy for her parents to accept the fact that they had to change their ways, but they understood that the future of their daughter was at stake and they decided to collaborate.

The first step was to write down what the family ate daily for a week, what Theresa ate at school, and the family's physical activity. From there we started introducing healthy changes and substituting other options for their greasy, sugary, heavy-calorie meals.

Aside from these changes in diet, Theresa and her parents, along with her younger sister, started organizing family activities that involved physical exercise, from visiting the national parks to going for a walk every day after dinner.

Theresa's communication with her family improved a lot. They were able to understand the loneliness Theresa was feeling at school and give her all their support. They even considered going to family counseling. They praised Theresa's natural qualities, like her drawing and musical skills and they even encouraged her to take some salsa classes, which she did. All of this helped Theresa to feel much better about herself. The bingeing and purging stopped. In a few months Theresa had gained enough self-esteem to be able to ignore the teasing at school. She was losing weight as a result of a balanced diet, and, most important, she understood the consequences that bulimia would have for her health.

It was not an easy road for Theresa and her family. There were lots of difficulties along the way, and more than once the old habits came back. But thanks to the support of her family, the pediatrician's help, and the guidance I was able to provide as a nutritionist, Theresa is today a healthy girl with a regular weight living in a much healthier family environment.

As you can see in the three cases we have explored, family cooperation was essential for recovery, no matter what the problem the child or adolescent was going through.

One of the best things parents can do for their children is to offer them a healthy diet from the time they are born. But remember also that it's never too late to start living healthily.

Appendix

Growth Charts

Birth to 36 months: Boys
Length-for-age and Weight-for-age percentiles

NAME _____

RECORD # _____

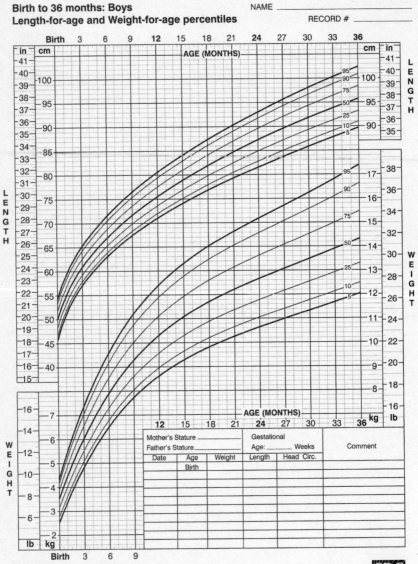

Published May 30, 2000 (modified 4/20/01).
SOURCE: Developed by the National Center for Health Statistics in collaboration with
the National Center for Chronic Disease Prevention and Health Promotion (2000).
http://www.cdc.gov/growthcharts

SAFER · HEALTHIER · PEOPLE™

Birth to 36 months: Girls
Length-for-age and Weight-for-age percentiles

NAME _____

RECORD # _____

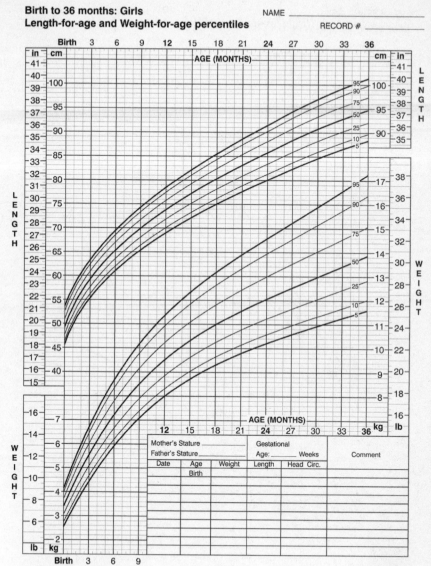

	Mother's Stature _____	Gestational	
	Father's Stature _____	Age: _____ Weeks	Comment
Date	Age	Weight	Length	Head Circ.	
	Birth				

Published May 30, 2000 (modified 4/20/01).
SOURCE: Developed by the National Center for Health Statistics in collaboration with
the National Center for Chronic Disease Prevention and Health Promotion (2000).
http://www.cdc.gov/growthcharts

SAFER · HEALTHIER · PEOPLE™

2 to 20 years: Boys
Stature-for-age and Weight-for-age percentiles

NAME _____

RECORD # _____

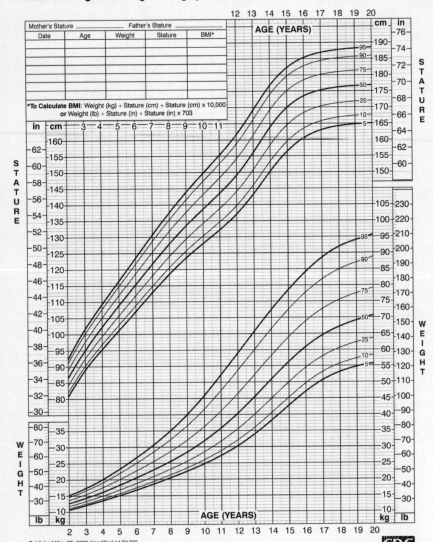

*To Calculate BMI: Weight (kg) ÷ Stature (cm) ÷ Stature (cm) x 10,000
or Weight (lb) ÷ Stature (in) ÷ Stature (in) x 703

Published May 30, 2000 (modified 11/21/00).
SOURCE: Developed by the National Center for Health Statistics in collaboration with
the National Center for Chronic Disease Prevention and Health Promotion (2000).
http://www.cdc.gov/growthcharts

CDC

SAFER · HEALTHIER · PEOPLE™

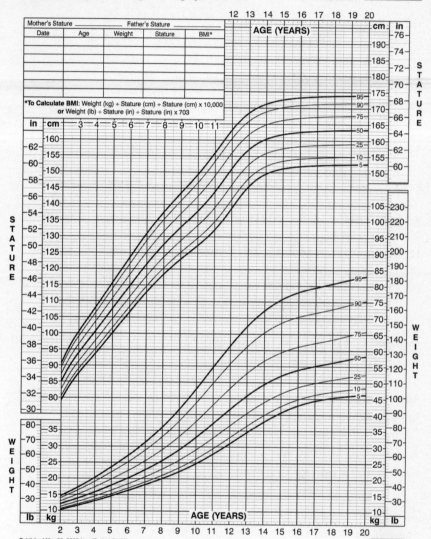

2 to 20 years: Girls
Stature-for-age and Weight-for-age percentiles

NAME _____

RECORD # _____

Published May 30, 2000 (modified 11/21/00).
SOURCE: Developed by the National Center for Health Statistics in collaboration with
the National Center for Chronic Disease Prevention and Health Promotion (2000).
http://www.cdc.gov/growthcharts

SAFER·HEALTHIER·PEOPLE™

Calorie Requirements for Children and Adolescents

Age group	Calories	Sedentary	Moderate	Active
2–3 years old	1,000–1,200 cal.	1,000 cal.	1,200 cal.	1,400 cal.
4–5 years old	1,300–1,400 cal.	1,200 cal.	1,400 cal.	1,600 cal.
6–8 years old	1,500–1,600 cal.	1,400 cal.	1,600 cal.	1,800 cal.
9–11 years old	1,600–1,800 cal.	1,600 cal.	1,800 cal.	2,000 cal.
12–15 years old	1,800–2,200 cal.	1,600 cal.	2,000 cal.	2,400 cal.
16–19 years old	2,200–2,600 cal.	1,800 cal.	2,400 cal.	2,800 cal.

Sedentary: Less than thirty minutes of moderate physical activity in addition to normal daily routine.

Moderately active: Thirty to sixty minutes of moderate physical activity in addition to normal daily routine.

Active: Sixty or more minutes of moderate to intense physical activity in addition to normal daily routine.

Water Needs for Children

There is no simple answer for how much water your child needs. Each person needs a different amount of water depending on how much water the body uses (based on body size and composition, activity level, and the temperature and humidity of the environment). But as a general rule, depending on the calorie intake of your child:

1,000 calorie daily intake = about 3 to 4 cups of water/fluids a day
1,500 calorie daily intake = about 4 to 6 cups of water/fluids a day
2,000 calorie daily intake = about 6 to 8 cups of water/fluids a day

The best advice for your children: "Drink water before feeling thirsty or when thirsty."

Resource Guide

In this section you will find telephone numbers and addresses for organizations and institutions that provide information or that will assist you in getting help to prevent or treat your child's obesity.

Besides the telephone numbers, you will also find Internet addresses for Web sites where you can access very valuable information. Even if you do not have a computer at home, you can always consult the Internet through a free connection at your local public library. Don't worry if you don't know how to use a computer, because the library staff will help you.

Where to Find a Doctor for Your Child

Community Health Centers
888-ASK-HRSA (800-275-4772)
www.bphc.hrsa.gov/databases/fqhc/
They provide medical attention to children and families without medical insurance, but whose annual income is too high to be admitted into federal

programs like Medicare. There are about three thousand community health centers through the fifty states and Puerto Rico.

To be treated, you only need to provide them with the number of members in your family and your income. The consultation will be free or at a very low cost, depending on your income. If for any reason the services don't fit your needs, they can help you to find some alternatives. To find a health center in your area, call the phone number that appears above. They can assist you in Spanish too.

You can also use the HRSA Web site (Health Resources and Service Administration, the federal office that provides this service), also noted above. Here all you need to do is insert your state and zip code and the health centers near you will appear. You just need to fill in your city, state, and zip code, and a list will appear with the health centers and their addresses. You don't need to give any other information because nearly all the clinics provide pediatric services, and in case they don't, they will direct you to one that does.

State Children's Health Insurance Program (SCHIP)
877-KIDS-NOW (877-543-7669)
www.insurekidsnow.gov/espanol/index.htm (Spanish)
www.insurekidsnow.gov (English)

This telephone number will connect you to a program in the state from which you are calling. It is a program that provides medical coverage for low-income babies and children.

When you call this number you will be assisted in Spanish, if you wish, and you can also get information from their Web site.

Medicaid
www.hcfa.gov/medicaid/obs5.htm (to find local phone numbers)
www.hcfa.gov/medicaid/stateplan/map.asp (requirements)

You can find the telephone number for Medicaid in your state in the government listings in the white pages of your phone book under "County Social Service Office."

Medicaid is a joint federal and state program where you can get free medical attention if you have an annual income below the limit determined by each state.

At the first Internet address above you will find the telephone number you can call in your state and the number where Spanish is spoken. On the second Web page given you will find the requirements in each state for you to be accepted to a Medicaid program, but it will be easier for someone to explain this to you by phone. If you want to learn more about Medicaid, this is a good source of information.

Programs Offering Help with Children's Nutrition

National School Lunch Program and School Breakfast Program
USDA
Food and Nutrition Service
Public Information Staff
3101 Park Center Drive, Room 914
Alexandria, VA 22302
(703-305-2062)
www.fns.usda.gov/cnd
The National School Lunch and Breakfast Program offers free or low-cost meals for children of low-income families. The meals are provided at public and private nonprofit schools and they comply with the federal Dietary Guidelines for Americans. Families with regular incomes can also participate in the program, paying full price for the meals.

For information on how the program works in your community you can call the number above or select "Contacts" at the Web site provided. You will find there the agency in your state that is responsible for the administration of the programs.

Women, Infants, and Children (WIC)
3101 Park Center Drive, Room 819
Alexandria, VA 22302
703-305-1747 (Spanish)
703-305-2747 (English)
www.fns.usda.gov/wic

This program provides food, nutrition advice, and help in finding prenatal attention for pregnant women, mothers (nursing or not), babies, and children up to five years old. WIC, which is what people call this program, provides coupons for free food that are accepted in certain authorized supermarkets. To be accepted into this program, your income must be below a predetermined level.

Organizations That Provide Information About Health Care

Su Familia
866-Su-Familia (866-783-2645)
Monday–Friday, 9:00 A.M. to 6:00 P.M. EST
Su Familia provides information on your options for obtaining medical insurance in your community. They will also answer questions regarding your health. The information is confidential and is offered both in Spanish and in English. They receive a lot of calls, so you may get an answering machine. If you leave your name and number, they will return your call.

The National Alliance for Hispanic Health
1501 Sixteenth Street, N.W.
Washington, DC 20036
202-387-5000
www.hispanichealth.org
The National Alliance for Hispanic Health is the organization that promotes the Su Familia information program, and here they will orient you on where and how you can get medical help.

National Committee for Quality Assurance
2000 L Street, N.W., Suite 500
Washington, DC 20036
888-275-7585
Monday–Friday, 8:30 A.M. to 5:30 A.M. EST
www.healthchoices.org

This is a nonprofit organization that analyzes insurance companies that provide information to the public. Through their Internet site you can see how your medical insurance is rated and/or what medical insurance is available in your area. On their Web pages you can look up medical insurance by state, by area code, or by company name.

Agency for Healthcare Research and Quality
2101 East Jefferson Street, Suite 501
Rockville, MD 20852
301-594-1364
www.ahcpr.gov/consumer/spchoos1.htm (Spanish)
www.ahcpr.gov/consumer/insuranc.htm (English)
AHRQ is a government agency that provides information about the quality of medical services given by different insurance companies. You can call their phone number to order a guide about the types of medical insurance on the market. There is a lot of information on their Web site, both in English and in Spanish, about how to choose a health plan or medical insurance.

National Association of Insurance Commissioners
www.naic.org/1regulator/usamap.htm
Every state has different regulations regarding the rules that medical insurance companies have to follow. On this organization's Web site there is a map of the United States. Here you can find a great deal of information regarding the regulations of medical insurance in your state.

Web Sites Where You Can Calculate
Your Child's Body Mass Index

www.niñoslatinossanos.com
www.healthylatinochildren.com
These are the two Web sites for this book, *Gordito Doesn't Mean Healthy*. Here you can calculate your child's body mass index automatically to find out if he or she is overweight or not. Furthermore, you'll find the Latino

food pyramid, comments from other parents who are facing the same problems as you, and information on how to create a healthier Latino lifestyle.

www.caloriecontrol.org/bmi.htm
Automatically calculates the body mass index and provides a chart with normal BMIs according to height.

www.thusness.com/bmi.t.html
Calculates the BMI in inches and pounds.

Information on Nutrition

American Dietetic Association
216 West Jackson Boulevard
Chicago, IL 60606-6995
Nutrition Hotline: 800-366-1655
www.eatright.org
With a phone call to this organization, you can get a recommendation for a nutritionist or a registered dietitian in your area. A registered nutritionist (designated by the initials RD after the name) is a person who has credentials in nutrition after passing an exam given by the Commission on Dietetics Registration.

5 a Day for Better Health Program
888-EAT-FIVE
www.5aday.gov
www.ca5aday.com (California)
The 5 a Day for Better Health Program is a national initiative to increase consumption of fruits and vegetables by all Americans to five to nine servings a day. The program provides consumers with specific information about how to include more servings of fruits and vegetables into their daily routines, and how to increase the availability of fruits and vegetables at home, school, work, and other places where food is served.

The 5 a Day program is the nation's largest public/private partnership for nutrition. The program includes federal, state, and local government agencies, industry, and volunteer organizations.

Food and Nutrition Service
U.S. Department of Agriculture
3101 Park Center Drive, Room 926
Alexandria, VA 22302-1594
703-305-2286
www.fns.usda.gov/fns/
The Food and Nutrition Service of the United States Department of Agriculture provides children and low-income families with food and nutrition education. This is where you will find several programs to help children, like the National School Lunch Program, the School Breakfast Program, the Summer Food Service, and other food programs for children and for adults also.

www.usda.gov
This is the official Web site of the United States Department of Agriculture, where you will find the latest nutritional guidelines, a food group pyramid, and further information about nutrition in Spanish.

www.mypyramid.gov
Here you will find an interactive system, where if you insert your age, sex, and level of physical activity, it will give you a list of the amounts and types of foods recommended for you weekly, following the government's pyramid.

Weight-Control Information Network
National Institutes of Diabetes and Digestive and Kidney Diseases
1 WIN Way
Bethesda, MD 20892-3665
800-WIN-8098 (800-946-8098 or 877-946-4627)
202-828-1025
www.niddk.nih.gov/health/nutrit/win.htm
This institution was created to provide scientific information about obesity, weight control, and nutrition, both to health professionals and to consumers. Among the publications dedicated to children there is a guide for adults to help overweight children and a workbook for adolescents.

Breastfeeding Help

La Leche League
1400 North Meacham Road
Schaumburg, IL 60173-4808
800-LA-LECHE (800-525-3243)
847-519-7730
www.lalecheleague.org/LangEspanol.html
This organization can answer all your questions about breastfeeding; they will give you advice on how to overcome the difficulties, and will put you in contact with groups of mothers in your area who can also help you. On their Web site they have a lot of information about lactation.

The National Women's Health Information Center
8550 Arlington Boulevard, Suite 300
Fairfax, VA 22031
800-944-WOMAN (800-994-9662)
www.4woman.gov
This is a government organization that provides information on many different health topics. They have a special advice line to give advice on breast feeding and referrals so you can find lactation consultants or lactation support groups in your area.

Information on Obesity

American Obesity Association
1250 24th Street, N.W., Suite 300
Washington, DC 20037
800-98-OBESE (800-986-2373)
www.obesity.org
If you call this number, they will provide you with important information on obesity. You can also calculate the body mass index here.

Information on Physical Activity

Centers for Disease Control and Prevention
1600 Clifton Road
Atlanta, GA 30333
404-639-3311
www.cdc.gov/spanish/verb/
This organization provides information about a governmental campaign promoting healthy habits among Latino families. On their Web site you will find information on nutrition, physical activity, and childhood obesity. It also offers a calendar where you will find events taking place in your community that you can enjoy with your family.

fitfamilyfitkids.com
This is a Web site sponsored by the Centers for Disease Control and Prevention. It has information about places available in your community where your child can get exercise. It also has information about nutrition and follows a few families, one of which is Latina, to see how they are coming along in making healthy changes in their lifestyles.

www.verbnow.com
This is a Web site targeting teenagers in their own language, to encourage them to exercise. It's a good place for your child to visit. It has video clips and all kinds of information and ideas about physical activity and nutrition for children and adolescents between the ages of nine and thirteen.

American Council on Exercise
4851 Paramount Drive
San Diego, CA 92123
800-825-3636
858-279-8227
www.acefitness.org
This nonprofit organization has an exercise program for children through which it provides information to parents about the type of physical activity recommended according to a child's age, and many other topics.

YMCA of the USA
101 North Wacker Drive
Chigaco, IL 60606
800-872-9622
312-977-0031
www.ymca.net
The YMCA has centers that offer all kinds of sports activities to men, women, and children, at reasonable prices. There are many centers all over the country, so it is very likely that there is one close to your home. The initials YMCA stand for Young Men's Christian Association. Many of these centers have pools with swimming programs and other sports for children.

American Alliance for Health, Physical Education, Recreation and Dance
1900 Association Drive
Reston, VA 20191-1598
703-476-3400
www.aahperd.org
This is an alliance of several associations that provide physical activity and a healthy lifestyle. It has a lot of information on all kinds of physical exercise programs for people of all ages.

Diabetes Help

American Diabetes Association
1701 North Beauregard Street
Alexandria, VA 22311
800-DIABETES (800-342-2383)
703-549-1500
www.diabetes.org
The American Diabetes Association is a nonprofit organization dedicated to research and information on this disease. By calling the toll-free number you can get information sent to you by mail about diabetes in children, as well as referrals to programs in your community for the treatment of diabetes in children and adults.

Children with Diabetes
5689 Chancery Place
Hamilton, OH 45011
www.childrenwithdiabetes.org
On this Web site you will find very complete information for children with diabetes and their families. Through this site you can sign up for a mailing list for families with diabetic children, in order to communicate with others in your situation.

National Council of La Raza
Center for Health Promotion
Chronic Disease Program
1111 Nineteenth Street, N.W., Suite 1000
Washington, DC 20036
202-785-1670
www.nclr.org
The National Council of La Raza is a nonprofit organization whose mission is to improve opportunities for Latinos. Within this organization there is a center for health promotion in which programs have been developed to treat chronic diseases like diabetes. If you call them, they can give you a good orientation regarding the programs that exist for diabetes and they'll give you information on nutrition and physical activity, if you want it. The National Council of La Raza publishes a storybook called *Day by Day with Auntie Betes* that explains how children can live their daily life with this disease.

National Information Center for Children and Youth with Disabilities
P.O. Box 1492
Washington, DC 20013-1492
(NICCHY)
800-695-0285
202-884-8200
www.nichcy.org (English)
www.nichcy.org/spanish.htm (Spanish)
There are several federal and state laws that protect children and adolescents with disabilities, including diabetes. Children with diabetes have full access

to public programs, including public schools and the majority of private schools. Students with disabilities have a right to accommodations and whatever changes are necessary in and around their schools in order to have the same access to education as the rest of the students. If you call NICCHY or go their Web page, they can give you information on the programs available in your state.

This organization will provide you with information both in English and Spanish on the laws dealing with disabilities, in order to ensure accommodation for your child's disease in school.

Questions About the Americans with Disabilities Act
800-514-0301
800-514-0383
www.usdoj.gov/crt/ada
The Americans with Disabilities Act is the law that protects children and adolescents with disabilities like diabetes. Here you will find more information about the law.

National Diabetes Education Program
1 Diabetes Way
Bethesda, MD 20892-3600
Telephone for ordering materials: 800-438-5383
www.ndep.nih.gov
This is a federal initiative with public and private members to improve the treatment of people with diabetes and for early detection. There is information for parents with diabetic children.

State Programs for Diabetes Control
www.cdc.gov/diabetes/states/index.htm
Through this Web site you can find state programs for the prevention and control of diabetes. You can get lists by state, by program name, or in alphabetical order. To obtain information on programs for children, you should contact the specific program in each state.

Meters for Testing Blood Sugar Without Pricking Fingers
Glucowatch: 866-459-2824; www.glucowatch.com

Soft-Tact: 866-763-8228; www.medisense.com
FreeStyle: 888-522-5226; www.therasense.com

Help and Information on Eating Disorders

Overeaters Anonymous
World Service Office
P.O. Box 44020
Rio Rancho, NM 87174-4020
505-891-2664
www.oa.org
Overeaters Anonymous is a nonprofit organization that helps people with eating disorders. This organization has thousands of free support groups all over the country. You can find a group close to you by calling the number above, or by checking their Web site.

National Association of Anorexia Nervosa and Associated Disorders
ANAD
P.O. Box 7
Highland Park, IL 60035
847-831-3438
Monday–Friday, 9: 00 A.M. to 5:00 P.M. CST
www.anad.org
This association will assist you by telephone and will give you information on how to find free support groups in your area as well as education about eating disorders.

National Eating Disorders Association
603 Stewart Street, Suite 803
Seattle, WA 98101
206-382-3587
800-931-2237
www.edap.org

Besides providing information, this organization will give you a list of treatment centers for eating disorders in children and adolescents.

Girl Power!
800-729-6686
www.health.org/gpower
This is a Web page in English for girls ages nine to thirteen with information and resources for healthy options. I highly recommend that your daughter visit this site.

Notes

CHAPTER 1

Page 2 *In fact, an obese child today has a 70 percent chance of being an obese*: United States Department of Human and Health Services. *Overweight in children and adolescents*. The Surgeon General's call to Action to prevent and decrease Overweight and Obesity. Dec. 2004.

Page 3 *For example, six out of every ten obese Latino children have type 2*:

Page 3 *According to a health and nutrition study carried out*: National Center for Health Statistics. "Prevalence of overweight among children and adolescents: United States, 1999–2002." NHANES 1999–2002, CDC.

Page 3 Obesity table. CDC, National Center for Health Statistics, National Health and Nutrition Examination Survey. Odgen et. al. *JAMA*. Sept. 15, 2004; 291: 2847–50.

Page 3 *A study comparing obesity rates among teenagers in fifteen industrialized countries*: Lissau, I., et al. "Body mass index and overweight in adolescents in thirteen European countries, Israel and the United States." *Archives of Pediatrics and Adolescent Medicine.* Jan. 2004; 158:27–33.

Page 5 *Scientists have proven children with a normal weight develop stronger immune*: Slobodianik, N. "Nutrientes e inmunidad." *Primeras Jornadas Internacionales de Nutrición, Inmunidad e Infección.* Buenos Aires, Argentina. 11, Apr. 12, 2003.

Page 6 *The idea that Latino parents believe that* gordito es saludable: Sanders, L., M.D., M.P.H. "Perception of obesity among parents of children attending preschool in the Miami community." Dyson Resident RFP, 2003 Symposium, La Jolla, California.

Crawford, Patricia B., Ph.D., R.D. "Perceptions of child weight and health in Hispanic parents: Implications for the California Fit WIC Childhood Obesity Prevention Project." The 129th Annual Meeting of APHA. October 2001.

Myers, S., and Vargas, Z. "Parental perceptions of the preschool obese child." *Pediatric Nursing.* Jan.–Feb. 2000; 26(1):23–30.

Alexander, M. A., et al. "Obesity in Mexican-American preschool children— a population group at risk." *Public Health Nursing.* Mar. 1991; 8(1):53–58.

Page 7 *Several studies over the past few years have shown a relationship between:* Baughcum, A. E., et al. "Maternal feeding practices and beliefs and their relationships to overweight in early childhood." *Journal of Developmental Behaviour of Pediatrics.* Dec. 2001; 22(6):391–408.

Spruijt-Metz, D., et al. "Relation between mothers' child-feeding practices and children's adiposity." *American Journal of Clinical Nutrition.* Mar. 2002; 75(3):581–86.

Birch, L. L. "Psychological influences on the childhood diet." *Journal of Nutrition.* Feb. 1998; 128(2 Suppl.):407S–410S.

Canetti, L., et al. "Food and emotion." *Behavioral Processes.* Nov. 2002; 60(2):157–64.

Page 7 *One study on this topic showed that immigrants begin*: Sanghavi, M., et al. "Obesity among U.S. immigrant subgroups by duration of residence." *The Journal of the American Medical Association.* 2004; 292:2860–67.

Dixon, L. B., et al. "Differences in energy, nutrient, and food intakes in a U.S. sample of Mexican-American women and men: Findings from the Third National Health and Nutrition Examination Survey, 1988–1994." *American Journal of Epidemiology.* Sept. 15, 2000; 152(6):548–57.

Page 9 *The first study to take a look at the genetic component of obesity*: Stunkard, A. J., et al. "The body-mass index of twins who have been reared apart." *New England Journal of Medicine.* May 24, 1990; 322(21):1483–87.

Page 9 *Today, there are many more studies that clearly show*: Ellis, L., and Haman, D. "Population increases in obesity appear to be partly due to genetics." *Journal of Biosocial Science.* Sept. 2004; 36(5):547–59.

Comuzzie, A. G. "The emerging pattern of the genetic contribution to human obesity." *Best Practice & Research Clinical Endocrinology & Metabolism.* Dec. 2002; 16(4):611–21.

Marti, A., et al. "Genes, lifestyles and obesity." *International Journal of Obesity Related Metabolic Disorders.* Nov. 2004; 28(3 Suppl.): 29S–36S.

Cai, G., et al. "Quantitative trait locus determining dietary macronutrient intakes is located on human chromosome 2p22." *American Journal of Clinical Nutrition.* Nov. 2004; 80(5):1410–4.

Page 9 *This connection between genes and obesity is even more pronounced*: Ayra, R., et al. "Evidence of a novel quantitative-trait locus for obesity on chromosome 4p in Mexican Americans." *American Journal of Human Genetics.* Feb. 2004; 74(2):272–82.

Comuzzie, A. G., et al. "The genetics of obesity in Mexican Americans: The evidence from genome scanning efforts in the San Antonio family heart study." *Human Biology.* Oct. 2003; 75(5):635–46.

Page 10 *According to a recent study done among obese pregnant mothers*: Whitaker, R. "Predicting preschooler obesity at birth: The role of maternal obesity in early pregnancy." *Pediatrics.* Jul. 2004; 114:29–36.

Page 11 *For example, scientists have discovered that certain rats that lack a particular gene*: April, D., et al. "Mice lacking the syndecan-3 gene are resistant to diet-induced obesity." *Journal of Clinical Investigation.* Nov. 1, 2004; 114(9):1354–60.

Page 12 *According to official statistics, one of every four Latino children*: National Center for Health Statistics, United States, 2004. Hyattsville, MD: Public Health Service. 2004.

Page 13 *Television is considered one of the main culprits of childhood obesity*: Andersen, R. E. "Relationship of physical activity and television watching with body weight and level of fatness among children." *The Journal of the American Medical Association.* Mar. 1998; 279:938–42.

Dennison, B. A. "Television viewing and television in bedroom associated with overweight risk among low-income preschool children." *Pediatrics.* Jun. 2002; 109:1028–35.

Page 14 *Also, nearly half of the Latino parents interviewed for one study said they felt more*: Duke, J., et al. "Physical Activity Levels Among Children Aged 9–13 Years—United States, 2002." Youth Media Campaign. National Center for Chronic Disease Prevention and Health Promotion, Centers for Disease Control and Prevention (CDC).

CHAPTER 2

Page 17 *. . . recent studies have shown obese children, especially obese Latino children*: Cruz, M. L. "The metabolic syndrome in overweight Hispanic youth and the role of insulin sensitivity." *Journal of Clinical Endocrinology and Metabolism.* Jan. 2004; 89(1):108–13.

Page 21 *In the case of Latinos, several studies have shown that some systems*: Arya, R., et al. "Factors of insulin resistance syndrome—related phenotypes are linked to genetic locations on chromosomes 6 and 7 in nondiabetic Mexican-Americans." *Diabetes.* Mar. 2002; 51(3): 841–47.

Page 22 *Several studies have shown that many Latino children are*: Goran, M. I. "Insulin resistance and associated compensatory responses in African-American and Hispanic children." *Diabetes Care.* Dec. 2002; 25(12):2184–90.

Goran, M. I., et al. "Impaired glucose tolerance and reduced beta-cell function in overweight Latino children with a positive family history for type 2 diabetes." *Journal of Clinical Endocrinology and Metabolism.* Jan. 2004; 89(1):108–13.

Page 25 *Research has shown that the earlier children go through this period*: Cole, T. J. "Children grow and horses race: Is the adiposity rebound a critical period for later obesity?" *BCM Pediatrics*. Mar. 12, 2004; 4(1):6.

Reilly, J. J. "Early life risk factors for obesity in childhood: Cohort study." *BJM*. Jun. 11, 2005; 330(7504):1357.

Skinner, J. D. "Predictors of children's body mass index: A longitudinal study of diet and growth in children aged 2–8 years." *International Journal of Obesity Related Metabolic Disorders*. Apr. 2004; 28(4):476–82.

Page 26 *Diabetes during pregnancy seems to be one of the factors*: Dietz, W. H., et al. "Periods of risk in childhood for the development of adult obesity—What do we need to learn?" *Journal of Nutrition*. Sept. 1997; 127(9):1884S–86S.

Page 26 *Also recent studies have shown that* where *a child accumulates*: Gillum, R. F. "Distribution of waist-to-hip ratio, other indices of body fat distribution and obesity associations with HDL cholesterol in children and young adults age 4–19 years: The Third National Health and Nutrition Examination Survey." *International Journal of Obesity Related Metabolic Disorders*. 1999; 23:556–63.

Cruz, M. L., et al. "Unique effect of visceral fat on insulin sensitivity in obese Hispanic children with a family history of type 2 diabetes." *Diabetes Care*. Sept. 2002; 25(9):1631–36.

Page 28 *Second, too much visceral fat is related to two illnesses that affect*: Cruz, M. L., et al. "Unique effect of visceral fat on insulin sensitivity in obese Hispanic children with a family history of type 2 diabetes." *Diabetes Care*. Sept. 2002; 25(9):1631–36.

Page 29 *Insulin resistance is hereditary, and not long ago*: Arya, R., et al. "Factors of insulin resistance syndrome—related phenotypes are linked to genetic locations on chromosomes 6 and 7 in nondiabetic Mexican-Americans." *Diabetes*. Mar. 2002; 51(3):841–47.

Page 29 *One study reports that one of every three obese Latino*: Goran, M. I. "Insulin resistance and associated compensatory responses in African-American and Hispanic children." *Diabetes Care*. Dec. 2002; 25(12):2184–90.

Page 31 *Nine of every ten obese Latino children who have parents*: Cruz, M. L. "The metabolic syndrome in overweight Hispanic youth and the role of insulin sensitivity." *Journal of Clinical Endocrinology & Metabolism*. Jan. 2004; 89(1):108–13.

Page 35 *Teenagers who don't think much of themselves are sadder*: Strauss, R. S. "Childhood obesity and self-esteem." *Pediatrics*. Jan. 2000; 105(1):e15.

Page 36 *In the case of Latino children, they're already*: Twenge, J. M. "Age, gender, race, socioeconomic status, and birth cohort differences on the children's depression inventory: A meta-analysis." *Journal of Abnormal Psychology*. Nov. 2002; 111(4):578–88.

Page 36 *The National Education Association conducted a study*: National Education Association. "Report on Discrimination Due to Physical Size." 1994; 11.

Page 37 *This phenomenon was proven in an interesting scientific*: Richardson, S. A., et al. "Cultural uniformity in reaction to physical disabilities." *American Sociological Review*. 1961; 241–47.

Page 37 *Participating in school sports*: Erkut, S. "Predicting adolescent self-esteem from participation in school sports among Latino subgroups." *Hispanic Journal of Behavioral Sciences*. Nov. 2002; 2(4):409–29.

Page 38 *People who develop type 2 diabetes during infancy*: Fagot-Campana, A. "Emergence of type 2 diabetes mellitus in children: Epidemiological evidence." *Journal of Pediatric Endocrinology & Metabolism*. 2000; 13(6 Suppl.): 1395–1402.

Page 38 *Teenagers who have a BMI higher than 75*: Kiess, W., et al. "Clinical aspects of obesity in childhood and adolescence." *Obesity Reviews*. Feb. 2001; 2(1):29–36.

Page 38 *People who have elevated levels of cholesterol as children*: Lauer, R. M. "Factors affecting the relationship between childhood and adult cholesterol levels: The Muscatine Study." *Pediatrics*. Sept. 1988; 82(3):309–18.

CHAPTER 4

Page 69 *In fact, there is evidence that dairy foods can keep adolescents from gaining*: Jacobsen, R., et al. "Effect of short-term high dietary calcium intake on 24-h energy expenditure, fat oxidation, and fecal fat excretion." *International Journal of Obesity*. 2005; 29:292–301.

Drapeau, G., et al. "Calcium intake and body composition in the Heritage Family Study." *Obesity Research*. 2003; 11(S):597–P.

CHAPTER 5

Page 97 *Some studies have looked into whether this phenomenon*: Kieffer, E. C. "Maternal obesity and glucose intolerance during pregnancy among Mexican-Americans." *Paediatric Perinatal Epidemiology*. Jan. 2000; 14(1):14–19.

Sowan, N. A. "Parental risk factors for infant obesity." *The American Journal of Maternal Child Nursing*. Sept./Oct. 2000; 25:234–41.

Page 98 *Study after study has shown that the most appropriate*: Howie, P. W., et al. "Protective effect of breast feeding against infection." *British Medical Journal*. Jan. 6, 1990; 300:11–16.

Lucas, A., and Cole, T. J. "Breast milk and neonatal necrotizing enterocolitis." *Lancet*. Dec. 22–29, 1990; 336:1519–23.

"Infant Feeding." Child Health USA 2002 Report. Maternal and Child Health Bureau.

Page 98 *But besides all this, there's another good reason to breastfeed*: Bergmann, K. E., Bergmann, R. L., von Kries, R., Böhm, O., Richter, R., Dudenhausen, J. W., and Wahn, U. "Early determinants of childhood overweight and adiposity in a birth cohort study: Role of breastfeeding." *International Journal of Obesity*. Feb. 2003; 27:162–72.

Dewey, K. G. "Is breastfeeding protective against child obesity?" *Journal of Human Lactation*. Feb. 2003; 19(1):9–18.

Page 99 *However, during the 1960s, the tendency to avoid breastfeeding started to change*: Wright, Anne L., and Schanler, Richard J. "The resurgence of breastfeeding at the end of the second millennium." *Journal of Nutrition*. Feb. 2001; 131:421S–25S.

Page 99 *In the past ten years, there's been a huge increase*: "Infant Feeding." Child Health USA 2002 Report. Maternal and Child Health Bureau.

Page 99 *We all know how much influence*: Sweeney, M., and Guilino, C. "The health belief model as an explanation for breastfeeding practices in a Hispanic population." *Advanced Nursing Science*. Jul. 1987; 9(4):35–50.

Samir, Arora, M.D., et al. "Major factors influencing breastfeeding rates: Mother's perception of father's attitude and milk supply." *Pediatrics*. Nov. 2000; 106(5):67.

Page 100 *Scientific studies have shown that this practice*: Armentia Alicia, M.D. *"Alergia a los inhibidores de a-Amilasa de cereales."* *Congreso de la Sociedad Española de Alergología e Inmunología Clínica*. Valladolid, Spain. 2002.

Page 101 *The study monitored babies between two and three days old*: Riordan, J. M., ARNP, Ed.D., FAAN, and Gill-Hopple, K., RNC, MSN. Sept. 26, 2002. Presentation at Wichita State University, Wichita, KS. "Testing relationships of breastmilk intake indicators with actual breastmilk intake."

Page 111 *Studies have shown that obese people have a difficult time*: Canetti, L., et al. "Food and emotion." *Behavioral Processes*. Nov. 2002; 60(2):157–64.

CHAPTER 6

Page 115 *According to one study, nearly three of every ten parents*: American Dietetic Association and Gerber Products Company. "Feeding Infants and Toddlers Study." *Journal of the American Dietetic Association*. Jan. 2004.

Page 115 *It's an appealing idea after weeks and months*: Macknin, M. L., et al. "Infant sleep and bedtime cereal." *American Journal of Disease in Childhood*. Sept. 1989; 143(9):1066–68.

Page 117 *According to a recent study, juices and sugared drinks*: American Dietetic Association and Gerber Products Company. "Feeding Infants and Toddlers Study." *Journal of the American Dietetic Association*, Jan. 2004.

Page 117 *Also, Latino children have more cavities*: Flores, G., Fuentes-Afflick, E., et al. "The health of Latino children: urgent priorities, unanswered questions and a research agenda." *Journal of the American Medical Association*. Jul. 3, 2002; 288(1):82–90.

Page 130 *According to a scientific study, children older than eighteen months who still feed*: Bonuck, K. A., and Kahn, R. "Prolonged bottle use and its association with iron deficiency anemia and overweight: A preliminary study." *Clinical Pediatrics*. Oct. 2003; 41(8):603–07.

CHAPTER 7

Page 136 *Different studies have shown that children between the ages of three*: Saariletho, S., et al. "Growth energy intake, and meal patterns in five-year-old children considered poor eaters." *Journal of Pediatrics*. Mar. 2004; 144(3):363–67.

Birch, L. L., and Deysher, M. "Caloric compensation and sensory specific satiety: Evidence for self-regulation of food intake by young children." *Appetite*. Dec. 1986; 7:323–31.

Page 136 *A study done on preschool children showed that overweight*: Birch, L. L., and Fisher, J. O. "Development of eating behaviors among children and adolescents." *Pediatrics*. Mar. 1998; 101:539–49.

Birch, L. L., et al. "The variability of young children's energy intake." *New England Journal of Medicine*. Jan. 1991; 324:232–37.

Page 136 *Let's say the parents are responsible for presenting*: Satter, E. *Child of Mine*. Palo Alto, CA: Bull Publishing, 1986.

Page 137 *Children will also learn to like foods that are presented*: Newman, J., and Taylor, A. "Effect of a means-end contingency on young children's food preferences." *Journal of Experimental Child Psychology*. Apr. 1992; 53(2):200–16.

Page 137 *You will have great influence over what foods your child*: Nicklas, T. A., et al. "Family and child-care provider influences on preschool children's fruit, juice and vegetable consumption." *Nutr Rev*. Jul. 2001; 59:224–35.

Page 138 *The sooner a child enters this phase, the greater*: Whitaker, R. C., et al. "Early adiposity rebound and the risk of adult obesity." *Pediatrics*. Mar. 1998; 101(3):E5.

Taylor, R. W., et al. "Rate of fat gain is faster in girls undergoing early adiposity rebound." *Obesity Research*. Aug. 2004; 12(8):1228–30.

Page 140 *One survey of Latino parents of preschool children showed*: Kaiser, L., et al. "Child feeding strategies in low-income Latino households: Focus groups observations." University of California, Davis. *Journal of the American Dietetic Association*. May 1999; 99(5):601–3.

Page 140 *One survey found that parents need to offer their children*: Birch, L. L., et al. "I don't like it; I never tried it: effects of exposure on two-year-old children's food preferences." *Appetite.* 1982; 3:353–60.

Page 142 *According to a study, children at this age who drink more*: Marshal, T. A., et al. "Diet quality in young children is influenced by peer-age consumption." *Journal of the American College of Nutrition.* Feb. 2005; 24(1):65–75.

Page 148 *Iron-deficiency anemia is common among preschool children and among*: Zive, M. M., et al. "Vitamin and mineral intakes of Anglo Americans and Mexican-American preschoolers." *Journal of the American Dietetic Association.* Mar. 1995; 95(3):329–35.

Page 148 *Also, studies have made a connection between obesity*: Nead, K. G., et al. "Overweight children and adolescents: A risk group for iron deficiency." *Pediatrics.* Jul. 2004; 114(1):104–8.

Page 148 *The same thing happens with zinc*: Zive, M. M., et al. "Vitamin and mineral intakes of Anglo-Americans and Mexican-American preschoolers." *Journal of the American Dietetic Association.* Mar. 1995; 95(3):329–35.

Page 149 *According to one study, Latina preschool*: Ibid.

Page 149 *Fifty years ago, orange juice was the number one*: Dennison, B. A. "Fruit juice consumption by infants and children: A review." *Journal of the American College of Nutrition.* Oct. 1996; 15(5 Suppl.):4S–11S.

Page 151 *One last appeal for the family meal: Children who eat*: Gillman, M. W., et al. "Family dinner and diet quality among older children and adolescents." *Archives of Family Medicine.* Mar. 2000; 9:235–40.

CHAPTER 8

Page 161 *There are two factors, according to a number of studies, that contribute to obesity*: Giammattei, J., et al. "Television watching and soft drink consumption." *Archives of Pediatric & Adolescent Medicine.* Sept. 2003; 157:882–86.

Ariza, A. J., et al. "Risk factors for overweight in five- to six-year-old Hispanic-American children: A pilot study." *Journal of Urban Health.* Mar. 2004; 81(1):150–61.

Page 164 *According to one study, children who eat at the table with their families*: Gillman, M. W., et al. "Family dinner and diet quality among older children and adolescents." *Archives of Family Medicine*. Mar. 2000; 9(3):235–40.

Page 165 *It is fully demonstrated that children who eat a good breakfast*: Kleinman, R. E., et al. "Diet, breakfast, and academic performance in children." *Annals of Nutrition and Metabolism*. 2002; 46(1 Suppl.):24–30.

Nicklas, T. A., et al. "Breakfast consumption affects adequacy of total daily intake in children." *Journal of American Dietetic Association*. Aug. 1993; 93:886–91.

Page 168 *According to another study, children who have the option*: Cullen, K. W., et al. "Effect of a la carte and snack bar foods at school on children's lunchtime intake of fruits and vegetables." *Journal of American Dietetic Association*. Dec. 2000; 100(12):1482–86.

Page 178 French, S. A., et al. "National trends in soft drink consumption among children and adolescents age 6 to 17 years: prevalence, amounts and sources, 1977/1978 to 1994/1998." *Journal of American Dietetic Association*. Oct. 2003; 103(10):1326–31.

Page 178–79 *A study done on the consumption of soda by children between the ages of nine and fourteen*: Berkey, C. S., et al. "Sugar-added beverages and adolescent weight change." *Obesity Research*. May 2004; 12(5):778–88.

Page 179 *This was shown in a study that followed the habits of schoolchildren*: Blum, J. W. "Beverage consumption patterns in elementary school-aged children across a two-year period." *Journal of the American College of Nutrition*. Apr. 2005; 24(2):93–98.

Page 179 *. . . in addition to the fact that they ran more risk of becoming overweight*: Harnack, L., et al. "Soft drink consumption among U.S. children and adolescents: Nutritional consequences." *Journal of the American College of Nutrition*. Apr. 1999; 99(4):436–41.

Page 179 *There is research that links teenage fractures to sodas*: Wyshak, G. "Teenaged girls, carbonate beverage consumption and bone fractures." *Archives of Pediatric & Adolescent Medicine*. Jun. 2000; 154(6):610–13.

Page 179 *Finally, an added problem regarding drinking sweetened soda is a marked*: Marshall, T. A., et al. "Dental cavities and beverage consumption in young children." *Pediatrics*. Sept. 2003; 112(3 Pt 1):e184–91.

Page 179 *The American Academy of Pediatrics has recently expressed concern*: American Academy of Pediatrics Committee on School Health. "Soft drinks in schools." *Pediatrics*. Jan. 2004; 113(1 Pt 1):152–54.

Page 179 *But besides school, one of the other places where children tend*: Grimm, G. C., et al. "Factors associated with soft drink consumption in school-aged children." *Journal of the American Dietetic Association*. Aug. 2004; 104(8):1244–49.

Giammattei, J., et al. "Television watching and soft drink consumption: Associations with obesity in 11- to 13-year-old schoolchildren." *Archives of Pediatric & Adolescent Medicine*. Sept. 2003; 157(9):882–86.

Page 181 *There are a number of studies that link the number of hours*: Proctor, M. H., et al. "Television viewing and change in body fat from preschool to early adolescence: The Framingham Children's Study." *International Journal of Obesity*. Jul. 2003; 27:827–33.

Page 181 *These ads influence the kind of foods that children will eat later*: Kotz, K., and Story, M. "Food advertisements during children's Saturday morning television programming: Are they consistent with dietary recommendations?" *Journal of the American Dietetic Association*. Nov. 1994; 94(11):1296–1300.

Coon, K. A., and Tucker, K. L. "Television and children's consumption patterns: A review of the literature." *Minerva Pediatrics*. Oct. 2002; 54(5):423–36.

Page 181 *Latino children are the ones who watch more television during*: "America after 3 PM: A Household Survey on Afterschool in America." EP Afterschool Alliance.

Page 182 *Having a television in a child's room is linked to obesity*: Dennison, B. A., et al. "Television viewing and television in bedroom associated with overweight risk among low-income preschool children." *Pediatrics*. Jun. 2002; 109(6):1028–35.

Page 190 *But research shows that you get far better results by not forcefully*: Birch, L. L., and Davison, K. K. "Family environmental factors influencing the developing behavioral controls of food intake and childhood overweight." *Pediatric Clinics of North America.* Aug. 2001; 48(4):893–907.

Page **193** *According to a recent study, many Latino parents cannot do this*: "Physical activity levels among children aged 9–13 years." *Morbidity and Mortality Weekly Report.* Centers for Disease Control and Prevention. Aug. 22, 2003; 52(33):785–88.

Page **195** *It is shown that just cutting the hours your child spends watching television*: Epstein, L. H., et al. "Decreasing sedentary behaviors in treating pediatric obesity." *Archives of Pediatrics & Adolescent Medicine.* Mar. 2000; 154(3):220–26.

CHAPTER 9

Page **196** *"Adolesence is a crucial stage in life"*: www.adolescentesxlavida. com.ar

Page **197** *Adolescence is the last critical stage in the development of obesity*: Dietz, W. H. "Periods of risk in childhood for the development of adut obesity—What do we need to learn?" *Journal of Nutrition.* Sept. 1997; 127(9):1884S–86S.

Page **197** *The type of obesity that develops or persists during adolescence*: Dietz, W. H. "Childhood weight affects adult morbidity and mortality." *Journal of Nutrition.* Feb. 1998; 128(2 Suppl.):411S–14S.

Guo, S. S., et al. "Predicting overweight and obesity in adulthood from body mass index values in childhood and adolescence." *American Journal of Clinical Nutrition.* Sept. 2002; 76(3):653–58.

Page **197** *Obese teenagers are much more likely to become obese adults*: Gordon-Larsen, P., et al. "Five-year obesity incidence in the transition period between adolescence and adulthood: The National Longitudinal Study of Adolescent Health." *American Journal of Clinical Nutrition.* Sept. 2004; 80(3):569–75.

Page **199** *This isn't strange since according to one study, an adolescent's*: Cavadini, C., et al. "U.S. adolescent food intake trends from 1965 to 1996." *The Western Journal of Medicine.* Dec. 2001; 173(6):378–83.

Diehl, J. M. "Food preferences of 10- to 14-year-old boys and girls." *Schweiz Med Wochenschr.* Feb. 6, 1999; 129(5):151–61.

Page 200 *There are studies that show that when teenagers have the option*: Kubik, M. Y., et al. "The association of the school food environment with dietary behaviors of young adolescents." *American Journal of Public Health.* Jul. 2003; 93(7):1168–73.

Page 200 *Excessive teenage consumption of fast food is also related to having*: French, S. A. "Fast food restaurant use among adolescents: associations with nutrient intake, food choices and behavioral and psychosocial variables." *International Journal of Obesity and Related Metabolic Disorders.* Dec. 2001; 25(12):1823–33.

Page 201 *Investigators have detected that in Latino children, and especially in girls*: Novotny, R., et al. "Calcium intake of Asian, Hispanic and white youth." *Journal of the American College of Nutrition.* Feb. 2003; 22(1):64–70.

Page 201 *By the time children reach adolescence, they are drinking*: Murphy, M., et al. "Beverages as a source of energy and nutrients in diets of children and adolescents." *Experimental Biology.* 2005 Abstract 275.4.

Page 201 *An added problem in drinking less milk is that they can*: Gordon, M. "Prevalence of vitamin D deficiency among healthy adolescents." *Archives of Pediatric and Adolescent Medicine.* Jun. 2004; 158:531–37.

Page 201 *Latino children are the group with the most cavities in the United States*: Shenkin, J. D. "Soft drink consumption and cavities risk in children and adolescents." *Gen Dent.* Jan.–Feb. 2003; 51(1):30–36.

Page 202 *According to a study that followed more than 15,000 children*: Field, A. E. "Relation between dieting and weight change among preadolescents and adolescents." *Pediatrics.* 2003; 112(4):900–06.

Page 208 *Furthermore, recent studies have shown that people who*: Spiegel, K., et al. "Leptin levels are dependent on sleep duration: relationships with sympathovagal balance, carbohydrate regulation, cortisol, and thyrotropin." *Journal of Clinical Endocrinology and Metabolism.* Nov. 2004; 89(11):5762–71.

Taheri, S., et al. "Short sleep duration is associated with reduced leptin, elevated ghrelin, and increased body mass index." *PLoS Med.* Dec. 2004; 1(3):662.

Page 210 *As a matter of fact, Latino adolescents have the highest rate*: Centers for Disease Control and Prevention, National Center for Chronic Disease Prevention and Health Promotion, National Youth Risk Behavior Survey (YRBS). 2004.

Iachan, R., et al. "Prevalence of and risk factors for depressive symptoms among young adolescents." *Archives of Pediatrics and Adolescent Medicine*. Aug. 2004; 158(8).

Page 215 *It is a proven fact that overweight adolescents are more often*: Strauss, R. S., et al. "Social marginalization of overweight children." *Archives of Pediatrics and Adolescent Medicine*. Aug. 2003; 157:746–52.

Page 215 *Furthermore, adolescents who are the object of jokes and teasing*: Eisenberg, M. E. "Associations of weight-based teasing and emotional well-being among adolescents." *Archives of Pediatrics and Adolescent Medicine*. Aug. 2003; 157:733–738.

Page 217 *Insufficient physical exercise is the main cause of obesity in adolescents*: Patrick, K., et al. "Diet, physical activity and sedentary behaviors as risk factors for overweight adolescence." *Archives of Pediatric and Adolescent Medicine*. Apr. 2004; 158:385–90.

Page 217 *Encouraging your child to take part in physical activities*: Neumark-Sztainer, D., et al. "Factors associated with changes in physical activity." *Archives of Pediatric and Adolescent Medicine*. Aug. 2003; 157:803–10.

CHAPTER 10

Page 220 *But recent studies have shown that belief is wrong*: Kuba, S. A., and Harris, D. J. "Eating disturbances in women of color: An exploratory study of contextual factors in the development of disorders eating in Mexican-American women." *Health Care Women International*. Apr.–May 2001; 22(3):281–98.

Page 220 *Moreover, this eating disorder is the one that afflicts the most boys*: Field, A. E., et al. "Racial/ethnic and gender differences in concern with weight in bulimic behaviors in adolescents." *Obesity Research*. Sept. 1997; 5(5):447–54.

Page 225 *A recent study showed that genetics may play a role in anorexia*: Ribases, M., et al. "Association of BDNF with anorexia, bulimia and age onset of weight loss in six European populations." *Human Molecular Genetics.* Jun. 15, 2004; 13(12):1205–12.

Page 226 *However, some studies have shown that eating disorders affect*: Vander Wal, J.S. "Eating and body image concerns among average-weight and obese African-American and Hispanic girls." *Eating Behaviors.* May 2004; 5(2):181–87.

Page 226 *Surveys say Latina girls are more likely to be binge eaters*: Fitzgibbon, M.L., et al. "Correlates of binge eating in Hispanics, black and white women." *International Journal of Eating Disorders.* Jul. 1998; 24(1):43–52.

Page 226 *So when these Latina girls get to their teenage years*: "Shortchanging girls, shortchanging America." 1991; Washington, DC: American Association of University Women.

Page 227 *This stress is a big factor in developing eating disorders*: Perez, M., et al. "The role of acculturative stress and body dissatisfaction in predicting bulimic symptomatology across ethnic groups." *International Journal of Eating Disorders.* May 2002; 31(4):442–54.

CHAPTER 11

Page 230 *One recent study showed that even though overweight children want to lose the extra pounds*: Tyler, D.O. "Overweight and perceived health in Mexican-American children: A plot study in a central Texas community." *The Journal of School Nursing.* Oct. 2004; 20(5):285–92.

Page 233 *According to one study, 28 percent of overweight Latino children*: Goran, I. "Impaired glucose tolerance and reduced B-cell function in overweight Latino children with a positive family history for type 2 diabetes." *Journal of Clinical Endocrinology and Metabolism.* Jan. 2004; 89(1):207–12.

Page 239 *Today we know atherosclerosis begins in infancy and slowly gets*: Berenson, G.S., et al. "Association between multiple cardiovascular risk factors and atherosclerosis in children and young adults." *New England Journal of Medicine.* Jun. 1998; 338:1650–58.

Page 239 *Cholesterol levels during infancy are an important factor in determining the likelihood*: Lauer, R.M., et al. "Use of cholesterol measurements in childhood for prediction of adult hypercholesterolemia: The Muscatine Study." *The Journal of the American Medical Association*. Dec. 1990; 246:3034–38.

Page 240 Cholesterol chart: Treatment Recommendations of the National Cholesterol Education Program Report of the Expert Panel on Blood Cholesterol Levels in Children and Adolescents. *Pediatrics*. Mar. 1992; 89(Suppl.):525–84.

Page 240 *Nutritionists have proven that if children and teenagers follow a balanced diet with the appropriate number*: The Writing Group for the DISC Collaborative Research Group. "Efficacy and safety of lowering dietary intake of fat and cholesterol in children with elevated low-density lipoprotein cholesterol: The Dietary Intervention Study in Children (DISC)." *The Journal of the American Medical Association*. May 1995; 273:1429–35.

Page 243 *Latino children are more likely to suffer from this problem*: Hanevold, C., et al. "The effects of obesity, gender and ethnic group on left ventricular hypertrophy and geometry in hypertensive children: A collaborative study on the International Pediatric Hypertension Association." *Pediatrics*. Feb. 2004; 113(2):328–33.

Page 243 *Several studies have shown high blood pressure during infancy is a sure*: Lawlor, D.A., and Smith, G.D. "Early life determinants of adult blood pressure." *Current Opinion in Nephrology of Hypertension*. May 2005; 14(3):259–64.

Page 245 High Blood Pressure in Children Chart: Adapted from the National Heart, Lung and Blood Institute's Blood Pressure Tables for Children and Adolescents. May 2004.

Contact the Authors

You can send your comments to the authors at:
claudia@healthylatinochildren.com and
lourdes@healthylatinochildren.com.

Visit the book's Web site at www.healthylatinochildren.com, where you will find recipes, tips, and tools to help you plan your children's meals. Also, you will be able to share your experiences with other Latino parents.